healthy
diabetes

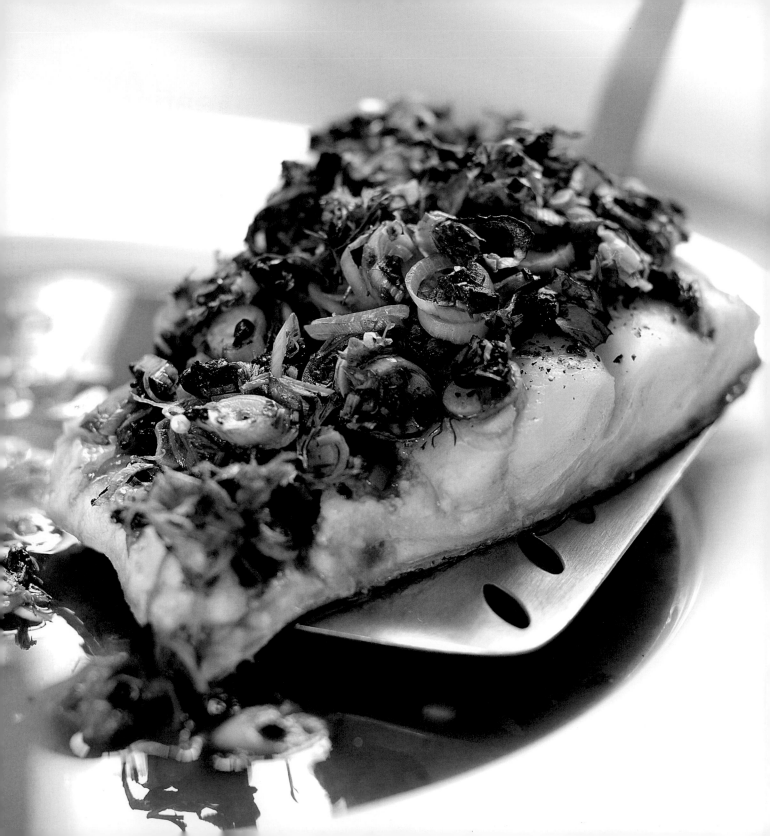

Antony Worrall Thompson with

Azmina Govindji BSc RD

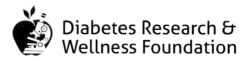
Diabetes Research &
Wellness Foundation

healthy eating for
diabetes

Photography by Steve Lee

Kyle Books

contents

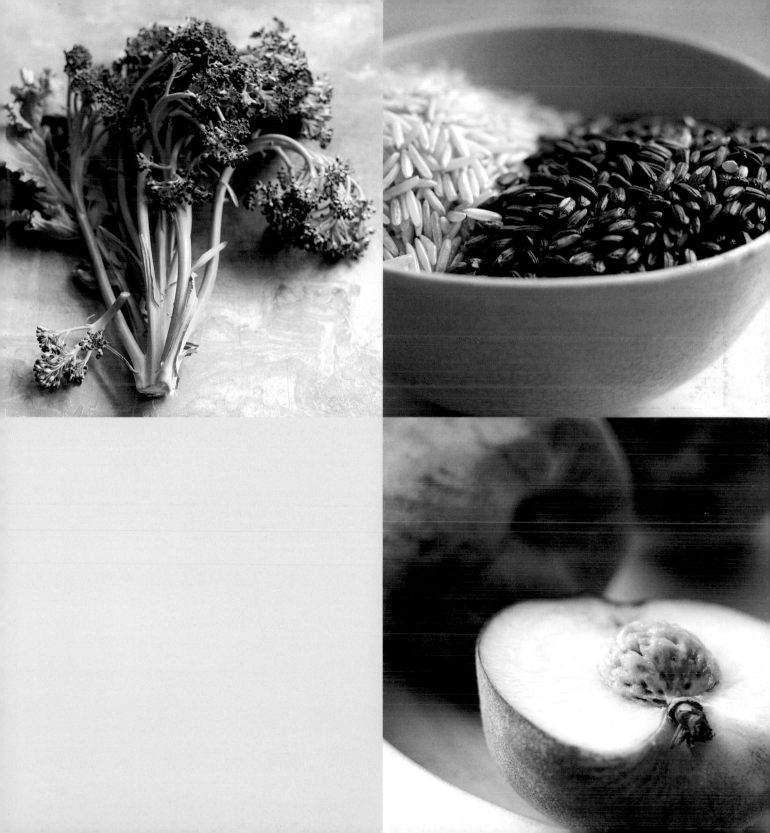

dedication

To Frank Shiel, my new Dad and father-in-law, who was recently diagnosed with diabetes.

There are too many people to thank, but certain individuals deserve a special mention:
To my wonderful wife, Jacinta and our two children, Toby and Billie, who suffered from my
lack of quality time yet supported me throughout as I managed to juggle my time through
3 books and everything else going on in my life.

To Louise, my energetic and ultra-efficient PA, who fielded hundreds of phone calls from
the publishers and who was regularly on hand to smooth troubled waters when the
pressures of deadlines occasionally took their toll.

To Fiona Lindsay, Linda Shanks and Lesley Turnbull at Limelight Management, who are
constantly there to make sure I have more than enough work to handle.

To my team at Notting Grill, especially David, George and Candido, who kept the boat
afloat in my often extended absences.

To the various friends Nicki, Kate, Sarah, Margot, Suzie, June, Anne and John, and Mike
and Nicky who acted unknowingly as guinea pigs for many of the recipes.

To Azmina Govindji, who waited patiently for the recipes so that she could nutritionally
analyse them and for producing an excellent section on the whys and wherefores of
diabetes, much of which I had limited knowledge of.

And finally to Muna Reyal, my editor and her fab team at Kyle Cathie for giving me
the opportunity to produce this cookbook. They turned my offerings into a beautifully
executed book that people with diabetes will find easy to understand and hopefully they
will realise life doesn't have to change that much when it comes to eating.

important note

The information and advice contained in this book are intended as a general guide to
healthy eating and are not specific to individuals or their particular circumstances. This
book is not intended to replace treatment by a qualified practitioner. Neither the authors
nor the publishers can be held responsible for claims arising from the inappropriate
use of any dietary regime. Do not attempt self-diagnosis or self-treatment for serious or
long-term conditions without consulting a medical professional or qualified practitioner.

foreword by Diabetes Research & Wellness Foundation

People often think that a diagnosis of diabetes means an end to enjoying their food and the beginning of a dull, uninspiring diet and special 'diabetic' foods. This definitely does not have to be the case. We have an abundance of fresh ingredients available to us; the influence of international cuisine; and a plethora of TV cookery shows and recipe books demonstrating that healthy eating can almost certainly be exciting and inspiring and joyous.

The Diabetes Research & Wellness Foundation (DRWF) is a registered national charity that supports vital diabetes research in the UK and around the world. Whilst doing so, the charity operates a Diabetes Wellness Network through which it provides NHS England Information Standard accredited information and educational support programmes to help people with diabetes establish and maintain good self-management skills. Promoting wellness and a better quality of life is central to our work. Our strapline of 'Staying well until a cure is found…' underpins the fundamental principle of our day-to-day support services. We know that supported self-management for people living with T1 and T2 diabetes is crucial to success and improved quality of life.

Azmina has been a valued contributor to DRWF publications for many years and sits on the charity's Editorial Advisory Board. She provides authoritative nutritional advice in a warm and wonderful way. She has performed many culinary demonstrations at DRWF events and supported individuals with diabetes in their 'healthy eating' learning. We are delighted to support this collaboration between Azmina and Antony which seeks to dispel the myth that the 'diabetic diet' is dull and boring. Their zest for life and food shall surely be an inspiring partnership.

We want everyone to know just how important healthy eating is and how easy it can be to create exciting, nutritional dishes to enjoy every day. This book will make a great addition to anyone's cookery book collection and we are really looking forward to trying out some of the dishes.

For a FREE information pack about the Diabetes Wellness Network and the support that DRWF offers, please email enquiries@drwf.org.uk quoting HEFD16 or visit our website www.drwf.org.uk

Sarah Bone
Chief Executive
Diabetes Research & Wellness Foundation

 Diabetes Research & Wellness Foundation

DRWF is a registered charity in England & Wales no 1070607 and a company limited by guarantee no 3496304.
Footnote: DRWF has not had any involvement in the editorial content of this publication.

what is diabetes?

Have you been newly diagnosed with diabetes? Or does someone in the family have diabetes? If so, read on for some home truths on just what diabetes is and how to live with it and still enjoy a full and active life.

When you have diabetes, the amount of glucose (sugar) in your blood is too high because your body is unable to use it properly. A hormone called insulin helps glucose to enter the cells where it is used as fuel by your body. If there is not enough insulin, or if the insulin you have is not working properly, then glucose can build up in your blood as a result.

Types of diabetes

* Type 1 diabetes occurs when there is a severe lack of insulin in the body. It is treated by insulin injections and a healthy range of foods.

* Type 2 diabetes is the most common type, accounting for about 90 per cent of all people with diabetes, and most people with Type 2 are overweight. In type 2 diabetes the body can still make some insulin, but it is either not enough for its needs or the insulin does not work properly. It can be treated by a healthy diet alone, or by diet and tablets, or sometimes by diet and injectable therapies.

What causes diabetes?

There is no one cause of diabetes and it seems to be caused by a combination of genetic and environmental factors. We know that it runs in families and we also know that if you are overweight you are more likely to get type 2 diabetes. There is no cure for diabetes yet, and there is no such thing as mild diabetes. The main aim of treatment is to avoid 'highs' and 'lows' in your blood glucose level. Together with a healthy lifestyle, this will help to improve your well-being and protect against long-term damage to your eyes, kidneys, nerves and heart.

Knowing the tell-tale signs

One of the difficulties with diabetes is that you might actually be symptom-free (particularly if you have type 2). Many people are diagnosed only after a routine examination by their GP. So, if you think you may have diabetes (for example, if you have a family history or one or more of the risk factors below), a simple blood test can put your mind at ease. Spotting the condition early will mean that it can be treated appropriately, which could help delay the onset of long term problems.

What to look out for
If you notice any of the following it could be an indication that you have diabetes:

* increased thirst, especially for sweet drinks

* you go to the toilet a lot, especially at night

* you feel very tired

* you are losing weight unexpectedly

* itching of the genital organs or recurrent thrush

* blurred vision

The above symptoms are more characteristic of type 1 diabetes, which is easier to diagnose as the symptoms appear quite quickly and can be relieved with treatment. However, if you have type 2 diabetes, which is more common in people over forty, these symptoms may be less apparent or even non-existent.

Low blood glucose

The medical term for low blood glucose is 'hypoglycaemia', although it is more commonly referred to as a 'hypo'. It occurs when your blood glucose reading is less than 4mmol/l. This is typically most likely to occur in people who take insulin or sulfonylureas. It can be caused by:

* missing a meal or snack

* engaging in strenuous activity without enough food beforehand

* taking more tablets or injecting more insulin than is needed

* drinking alcohol on an empty stomach

* not having enough carbohydrates

Sometimes, however, there may be no obvious reason for a hypo. Signs and symptoms of a hypo vary, but the common ones are light-headedness, a faint feeling, sweating, shaking, hunger and confusion.

A hypo should be treated with 15–20g of fast-acting carbohydrate, such as taking five glucose tablets immediately to raise your blood glucose. You should wait 15 minutes and test again. If there is no change, take a further 15–20g of fast-acting carbohydrate. After this, a longer acting carbohydrate, such as a glass of milk and a slice of whole grain toast, a banana or breakfast cereal with milk can be taken.

Metabolic Syndrome

You may have heard about metabolic syndrome and wondered what it was. It sounds like something from a science-fiction movie but it actually refers to a collection of medical conditions. These include:

✳ central obesity, which means a waist measurement of more than 94cm for men (92cm for South Asian men as they have been found to be even more at risk) and more than 82cm in women

✳ poor blood glucose control

✳ high blood pressure

✳ abnormal blood fats including raised triglycerides and low HDL (the 'good' form of cholesterol – see page 16)

✳ 'sticky blood' with an increased tendency to form clots

A diagnosis of metabolic syndrome is reached when three or more of these conditions occur together. Each of them is an independent risk factor for heart disease and having more than one increases the risk considerably.

What causes it?

The prevalence of metabolic syndrome is increasing globally. There appears to be a genetic factor at work, so having a family member with metabolic syndrome increases your risk. Current thinking is that all the conditions associated with it arise from one main cause: insulin resistance (IR). IR is a reduced sensitivity in the tissues of the body to the action of circulating insulin. As a result, the pancreas reacts by trying to produce more insulin, leading to high circulating levels in the blood. If the insulin resistance becomes severe, type 2 diabetes can develop.

Metabolic syndrome is sometimes said to be 'silent' since most people who have it are unaware of it. Risk factors include obesity, a family history of type 2 diabetes and a history of diabetes during pregnancy.

What can you do if you have metabolic syndrome?

Research has shown that both insulin resistance and the symptoms of metabolic syndrome can be improved by lifestyle changes, including physical activity and healthy eating. There is some research to suggest that a diet based mainly on foods with a low glycaemic index (see page 13) may improve insulin sensitivity in people with type 2 diabetes, but their role in metabolic syndrome is not clear at present. The good news is that these approaches, if successfully adopted, are very effective in reducing the risk of heart disease and of developing type 2 diabetes.

Lifestyle Guidelines for metabolic syndrome

✳ Take regular physical exercise – activities such as brisk walking.

✳ Cut down on the amount of fat and replace saturated fat with mono and polyunsaturated fats from vegetable sources and fish.

✳ Choose starchy carbohydrate and fibre-rich foods, fruit and vegetables.

✳ Aim for a healthier body weight and waist size.

✳ Drink alcohol in moderation only.

✳ Don't smoke.

food facts

What you eat is the most important part of your diabetes treatment. Whether you need to take medication or not, the foods you choose and how often you eat have a significant impact on your blood glucose. What you eat also affects the amount of fat (like cholesterol) in your blood. If you have diabetes, you already have an increased risk of developing heart disease, so watching what you eat is particularly important. Insulin or tablets are not a substitute for a healthy diet.

There are lots of healthy eating tips in this book. It's a good idea to pick out the changes that you feel will easily fit into your lifestyle, choosing foods you enjoy. Don't think in terms of foods that you must or must not eat. Healthy eating is all about balance, not forcing yourself to eat foods you dislike.

A taste of the Mediterranean

The Mediterranean way of eating, with its abundance of olive oil, garlic, fish, nuts, fruit and vegetables, has been associated with a lower risk of conditions such as coronary heart disease and cancer, so incorporating foods from Mediterranean cuisine into the diet for diabetes makes sense. And the good news is that recent research supports the idea that eating the right types of fat may be more important than making your fat intake really low. It has been shown that the total amount of fat eaten by people who live in Mediterranean countries is actually quite high, but when you take a closer look, you see that it's high in monounsaturated oils (such as olive oil), and omega-3 fats (such as those found in oily fish).

Research suggests that eating one or two servings of oily fish (such as salmon, herring, mackerel and tuna) a day can significantly reduce your risks of heart disease, and it even benefits those people who have already suffered a heart attack. People in Mediterranean countries also eat more fruit and vegetables, so they benefit from a range of nutrients including vitamin C, fibre and potassium.

Starchy foods (carbs)

Starchy carbohydrate foods, or carbs, (such as bread, rice, pasta, cereals, chapatis and potatoes) are typically low in fat. Many recipes in this book contain pasta, which, when eaten in moderate amounts, is an excellent carb for people with diabetes. Carbs that contain fibre also tend to be more filling, and if they are cooked using healthier cooking methods as in this book, they can be helpful if you are trying to lose weight.

Wholegrain varieties of bread and cereals as well as the skin on potatoes are high in fibre. High-fibre starchy foods such as bran-based cereals and wholemeal bread contain insoluble fibre, and are especially useful in preventing constipation. A high-fibre diet is good for you, but remember that when you eat more fibre, it is important to drink more fluid. Try to drink at least six to eight cups of fluid each day.

Oat-based cereals like porridge and muesli, and vegetables such as beans and pulses, provide you with a type of fibre called soluble fibre. These foods tend to be more slowly absorbed than low fibre starchy foods and they can play a significant part in keeping your blood glucose within a healthy range.

Instant hot oat cereals do contain soluble fibre, but because the oats have been 'mashed up' they are less able to slow down the rise in blood glucose after meals. It is important to spread your intake of starchy foods evenly through the day and to eat regular meals. This helps to reduce fluctuations in your blood glucose levels.

Are carbs good, bad or ugly?

Flicking through a magazine or surfing online, it is neither unusual nor surprising to see many articles on the latest trend in carbohydrates, whether they're about gluten, bloating, dieting and so on. How are you to know what's best in the case of diabetes? And is all this conflicting advice, or do the experts agree?

Let's start with some basics. The chemical structure of carbohydrates affects how they are metabolised in your body. What are sometimes called sugary, simple or refined carbs are made up of short chains of sugar. Longer chains of sugar are often called starchy or complex carbohydrates. Sugar-rich carbs, especially if they're in liquid form, will be broken down more easily, so they are more likely to make your blood glucose rise quickly (think sugared water). Recent evidence suggests that wholegrain and less processed carbs (like porridge or brown pasta) are better for your health than sugar and processed carbs (like white rice or pasta). Less processed carbs often tend to have a lower GI (see page 13).

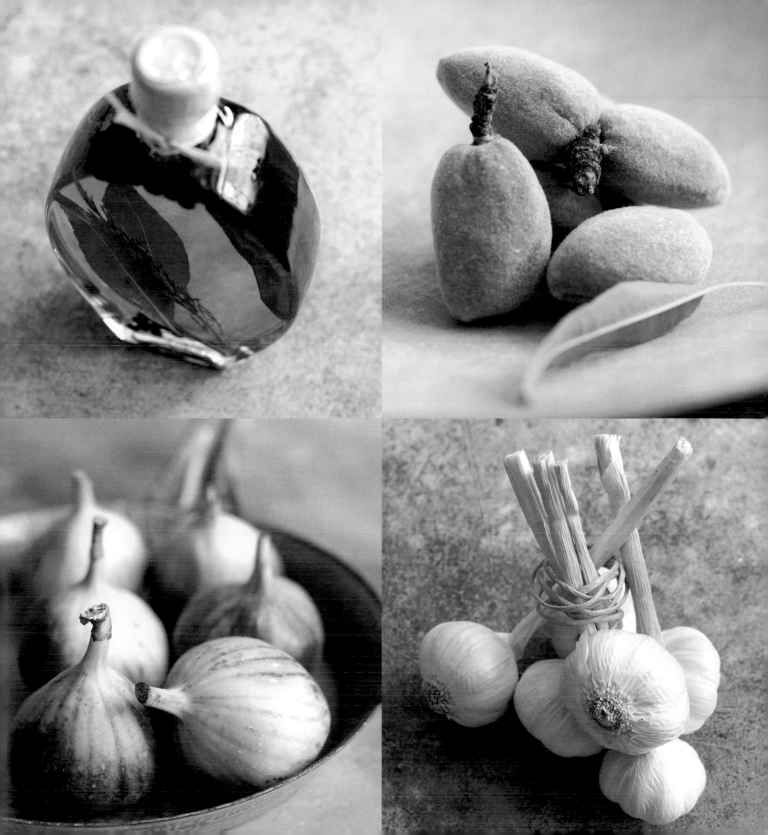

Examples of sugary carbs	Examples of starchy carbs	Examples of less processed starchy carbs
Glucose	Breads, including chapattis, pitta	Granary or seeded bread, wholemeal pitta, chapattis made from coarse wholemeal flour
Fructose, found in fruit, some vegetables and honey	Tortillas, etc.	
Sucrose, as in tabletop sugar	Pasta, noodles	Wholemeal tortilla
	Rice	Brown pasta
Maltose	Potatoes, plantains, cassava, yams	Brown rice
Lactose, found only in milk and milk products		Root vegetables cooked with the skin left on
	Cereals	Wholegrain cereals, porridge, bulgur wheat, quinoa

The low-carb way of eating

Low-carb diets, perhaps the best-known example of which is the Atkins diet, typically involve basing meals on meat, poultry, fish, eggs and cheese, whilst severely restricting all carbohydrate-rich foods such as bread, potatoes, pasta, rice, pizza, crisps, cereals and sugars. They also limit most fruits, some vegetables and many alcoholic drinks.

If you have diabetes and are thinking of lowering the amount of carbohydrate in your diet, you need to consider what medication you are on and seek medical advice – this is vital if you take insulin or drugs called sulphonylureas (gliclazide and glimperide are the most common).

Some advocates of low-carbohydrate diets suggest a moderate restriction can work, while others promote very low intakes to induce a condition known as ketosis. Ketosis is a state where the body switches from using sugars (glucose) to fats and ketones. This normally happens with long-term fasting and starvation, but can happen with very low intakes of carbohydrate. There is no evidence that being in ketosis has any advantages for people with diabetes. Ketosis is different for the ketoacidosis seen in uncontrolled type 1 diabetes where the body has very little or no insulin.

So, are there any benefits to be derived from reducing carbohydrate intake? It seems these are limited to the reduction in energy (calories) in the diet. It is simple maths – the reductions in energy intake seen in many studies of low-carbohydrate diets are often two to three times greater than those caused by low-fat diets. So, it appears that low-carbohydrate diets can work, and a number of people choose to try this approach and find it effective.

However, the reason it works is perhaps more simple than many an internet expert might have you believe. Note that some low-carb diets can encourage the complete omission of whole food groups, e.g. cereals, dairy products and fruit. Whilst some of these foods can be replaced by others and still provide the necessary balance of vitamins and minerals, professional advice from a dietitian is recommended to help minimise the risk of a nutritionally indequate diet.

Are some carbs better than others?

So, is pasta in or out? Should you be giving potatoes a miss? Meals are best tailored to the individual, rather than everyone aiming for the same goals, as some people will do better on fewer carbs than others.

Most people with type 2 diabetes would benefit from losing weight, so filling up on lots of high calorie carbs is unhelpful. If balanced meals and snacks are maintained, there's no reason why your favourite carbs cannot be a part of your daily menu. In fact, there are some carbohydrates that are actively encouraged – those with a low glycaemic index (GI; see opposite). Although recent evidence suggests that low GI diets are not effective in type 1 diabetes, diabetes organisations around the world (Diabetes UK, Canadian Diabetes Association, American Diabetes Association, Australian Diabetes Association) recommend the inclusion of low GI foods for helping to

Examples of Low-GI foods	Examples of Medium-GI foods	Examples of High-GI foods
Muesli and porridge	Beetroot	Bagels
Multi-grain and rye bread	Basmati rice	White and wholemeal bread
Fruit loaf	Potatoes, boiled	Water biscuits
Pasta	Rich tea biscuits	Glucose drinks
Baked beans	Pitta bread	Corn chips (tortilla crisps)
Lentils	Wheat biscuit cereals	Corn flakes
Apples, oranges and pears	Couscous	Puffed wheat
Yogurt	Ice cream	Puffed rice
Sweetcorn	Digestive biscuits	Sugar-rich breakfast cereals
Some high-bran cereals	Honey	Sports drinks
		Waffles

even out blood glucose levels in Type 2. However, the amount of carbohydrate you eat has a bigger effect on blood glucose than GI alone.

When it comes to sugar, which is also a carbohydrate food, the advice is different, but again, forget the myth that you can't have any sweet tastes in diabetes – see page 14 for more on sugar.

Glycaemic index (GI)

When you eat carbohydrate foods (such as bread, potatoes, pasta or cereals), the body digests the starch until, eventually, it becomes glucose (sugar). This can then be used by the body for energy and it is this glucose which contributes to the glucose levels in your blood.

Glucose also comes from other foods, but mainly from the starchy and sugary foods. So, is it as simple as just watching the starch and sugar in your diet?

Research shows that not all carbohydrate foods have the same effect on blood glucose. Furthermore, the amount and type of fat, the type of fibre and even the way food is cooked is important.

The GI is a ranking of foods relating to how these foods affect blood glucose levels. The faster a food is broken down during digestion, the quicker will be the rise in blood glucose. Since one of the main aims of treatment of diabetes is to keep blood glucose levels steady throughout the day, foods which cause sharp rises are best kept to a minimum, except in special circumstances, such as illness, hypoglycaemia (see page 8) or exercise. Foods that cause a rapid rise in blood glucose will have a high GI, so the key is to choose more low-GI foods regularly. The effect of a low-GI meal can run into the following meal, which helps to keep blood glucose more even throughout the day.

Since low-GI foods reduce the peaks in blood glucose that often follow a meal, they may have a role in helping to prevent or reduce the risk of getting type 2 diabetes if you are at risk, as in metabolic syndrome (see page 9). Some studies suggest that low-GI foods can help you to eat less as you feel fuller for longer. Research has also shown that people who follow an overall low-GI diet have a lower incidence of heart disease and lower-GI diets have also been associated with improved levels of 'good' cholesterol (see page 16).

Which foods should you go for?

'Whole' foods, such as wholegrains, and those high in soluble fibre, for example kidney beans or chickpeas, will take longer to be broken down by the body and will thus cause a slower rise in blood glucose. If you imagine how easy it is to digest puréed pea soup which is already in small pieces, it would make sense to suggest that the body doesn't need to mash this up for too long before it is ready to enter the bloodstream as glucose. Now imagine how much longer it would take to digest whole peas. The body needs to break down the skin of the peas before it even reaches the pulp, then it needs to break that down into a mush before it is small enough to enter the bloodstream. Whole peas will therefore make the blood glucose rise more slowly than the puréed soup. This is the case with most foods. Compare hummus to a whole chickpea casserole, mashed potatoes to a jacket potato and wholemeal bread to seeded bread.

Look at the whole food

It's important to know that not all low- or medium-GI foods are recommended for good health. The addition of fat and protein, for example, slows down the absorption of carbohydrate, giving foods a lower GI, so that chocolate, for instance, has a medium GI because of its fat content. And crisps and chips actually have a lower GI than potatoes cooked without fat. Milk and other dairy products have a low GI because of their high protein content, and the fact that they contain fat. So, if you choose only low-GI foods, your diet could be unbalanced and high in fat, which could lead to weight gain and an increased risk of heart disease. Overall balance is, then, the key to healthy eating and the right mix of foods will not only ensure better control of your blood glucose, but will also help you to obtain the wide variety of nutrients needed for good health.

The table above gives a comparison of the GI levels of various foods. The GI of a food only tells you how quickly or slowly it raises the blood glucose when the food is eaten on its own, so you need to bear in mind that in practice we generally eat foods in combination: bread is usually eaten with butter or margarine; potatoes are often eaten with meat and vegetables, etc. Cutting out all high-GI foods is not the answer; instead include more low-GI foods to lower the overall GI.

Eating a large portion of a low-GI food, like pasta, will increase its glycaemic load– this can make your blood glucose rise quickly, even though you chose a low-GI option. In general, you may find it easier just to remember that whole grains or unprocessed foods are likely to have a better effect on your blood glucose levels than processed or refined carbs. It's important to keep an eye on your portion sizes of all carbs, whether you think they're healthy or not.

The truth about sugar

Sugar is just calories; it has no benefits in terms of vitamins, minerals, protein or any other nutrient. However, we cannot ignore the fact that sugary foods taste good!

We all know that, whether you have diabetes or not, eating too many sugar-rich foods and drinks is not recommended for good overall health. Recently, there has been more emphasis on sugar and how it affects risks of

obesity, dental decay and even type 2 diabetes. Here we summarise the key recommendations from the recent UK government report on sugar and carbohydrates, and offer practical tips on how to enjoy small amounts of sugar-containing foods as part of an overall healthy eating plan.

The SACN Sugar and Carbohydrates Report
In July 2015, the Government's Scientific Advisory Committee on Nutrition (SACN)

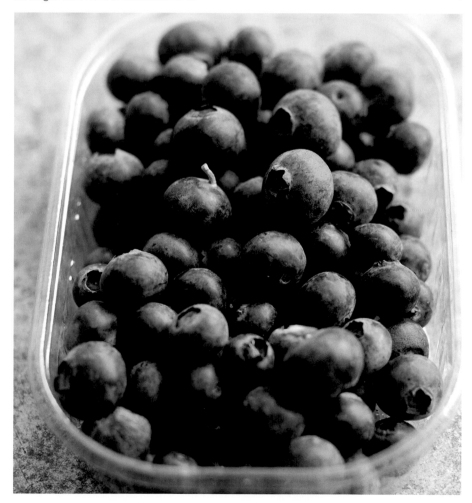

published an extensive review of the science on carbohydrate and made recommendations on how people should improve their diets so as to have a better balance of carbohydrate foods, especially sugar. Here are some key points:

* We are advised to drastically reduce our intake of what are called 'free sugars', by cutting total energy intake in half from 10% to 5%   e.g. cutting recommendations from 12–16 teaspoons per day in adult men and women to 6 8 teaspoons per day.

* This refers to sugar that is physically added to food by you at home or by manufacturers of food products, as well as sugars that are naturally present in honey, syrups and unsweetened fruit juices. Free sugars should count for no more than 5% of our daily energy (calorie) intake. We're currently having about 12% of our calories from sugars (teenagers have about 15%).

* We need to eat more fibre. The target to aim for is 30g a day; currently we're eating about 18g.

* The amount of carbs we eat in a day should remain the same as previous recommendations – 50% of our daily calories should come from starchy carbs, with particular emphasis on whole grains.

Why so much emphasis on sugar?
The review of the research by SACN showed that having too much sugar puts you at greater risk of tooth decay, and that there is an association between a high intake of sugars and a higher calorie intake, which increases risks of obesity. Sugar sweetened beverages (sugar-rich drinks) in particular were shown to increase Body Mass Index (BMI) in teenagers – this age group tends to drink the highest volume of sugar sweetened beverages.

There is also some research that suggests that having too many sugar sweetened beverages increases the risk of type 2 diabetes.

Helping to make sense of sugars
When you look at the National Diet and Nutrition Surveys (NDNS) that are carried out in the UK, you notice that we appear to be eating more free sugars and less fibre than the original targets before the SACN Report – they were 10 per cent energy from sugars and 24g fibre in a day. So, achieving the stricter targets will be a significant challenge. What you need to remember is that these are targets for the population, and each person can make changes towards these goals.

How do you know when sugar has been added? Of course seeing sugar on a food label is a dead giveaway, but note that sugar comes in different guises – it may be called dextrose, glucose, maltose, treacle, syrups, molasses, demerara, etc. Sugars that are naturally present in milk (lactose) and fruit (fructose) are not free sugars. Currently, there is no way of seeing the quantity of free sugars in a food, as labels only tell you the 'total sugars'. So, when you look at a label of a yogurt, for example, some of it will be free (added) and some will be lactose (milk sugar). Try to consider the whole food – does the food give you some goodness? In the case of a yogurt, it certainly gives you protein and calcium. And there are low fat, lower sugar types available that help you cut free sugars, saturated fat and calories.

Desserts
Having diabetes does not mean saying goodbye to desserts. All sorts of sweets and puddings can be incorporated into your diet, particularly if you choose appropriate ingredients. Half-fat creams, low-fat instant dessert mixes, fresh and dried fruit can all help to reduce the fat and sugar content of traditional puddings. To make your desserts even lower in fat, try using virtually fat-free fromage frais or low-fat natural yogurt. Base desserts on fruit as often as possible. The tempting recipes in this book will give you inspiration for sweet treats.

Sweeteners
Artificial sweeteners made from aspartame, saccharin and acesulfame potassium are sugar-free and will not cause a rise in your blood glucose levels. They may be used to sweeten foods but it is generally best to add them after cooking or in recipes that don't need to be heated as some people find they taste bitter when heated to high temperatures.

Sucralose, which has been made from sugar and processed so that it becomes sweeter than sugar without the calories, does not affect your blood glucose levels when eaten in normal amounts. Stevia comes from the stevia plant, and is 200 300 times sweeter than sugar. Both of these can be used in cooking and baking.

It's all a matter of personal choice. If you prefer to use a sugar substitute, this can be useful, for example, in cereals and desserts. This can help you cut your calories. However, if you prefer to use a little sugar, ensure that the other foods in your meal are nutritious by including, for instance, high-fibre cereal (such as porridge) for breakfast, beans and pulses in your main meals and fruit as the basis of desserts.

Fats

Advice given about fats can often sound confusing. If fats are so bad for you, how come some are essential? If spreading fats are better than hard fats like butter, why the caution with 'trans' fats in margarine? If a high blood cholesterol is unhealthy, how is it that foods which are high in cholesterol are not necessarily bad for you? One of the key tips for eating well, whether you have diabetes or not, is to choose healthy fats within an overall balanced eating plan.

The science behind cholesterol

Blood is delivered to the heart via the coronary arteries. As you get older, it is normal for these arteries to narrow, primarily as a result of Western lifestyle and food habits, which cause fatty deposits (atheroma) to be laid down within the artery walls. The fat then hardens (atherosclerosis), resulting in the reduction of the rate of blood flow. Also,

it is likely that the hardened fat becomes damaged and blood cells form a clot as a means of protection. A large clot can block the artery completely, causing a heart attack. If your blood cholesterol is high, you are more likely to develop atherosclerosis.

Fat is transported around the blood as lipids, which are carried in tiny particles called lipoproteins. Although having high blood cholesterol increases your chances of having a heart attack, some blood cholesterol is not harmful at all. Often termed 'good' cholesterol, high-density lipoprotein (HDL) represents the cholesterol which is being taken away from the body tissues back to the liver. Most of your cholesterol is, however, carried in the low-density lipoprotein (LDL) or 'bad' cholesterol. A high LDL level can increase your risk of a heart attack as it leads to the formation of fatty deposits in the arteries.

Therefore, the higher your HDL, the lower your risk of heart disease.

Is fat good or bad?

Fat has received a lot of attention recently. This was partly led by a number of articles in professional journals suggesting that saturated fats may not be the dietary villains we once suspected. Although there is clear evidence that a number of saturated fats increase cholesterol, the link between saturated fats doesn't appear to be quite as strong as previously thought. This is partly because some of the faults and weakness in the studies, which can lead to confusing results.

There are examples of types of fats opposite, but you may be familiar with the fact that saturated fats mainly come from animal fats (like fatty meat) and full-fat dairy products. The key message is not just about reducing saturated fat – it is about what that fat is replaced with. So,

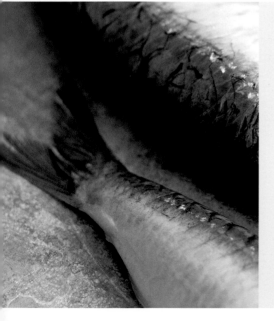

Did you know?

∗ Fat, weight for weight, provides twice the calories of starch, sugar or protein.
∗ Foods high in fat tend to be high in calories and are often also high in sugar.
∗ Essential fats are needed regularly in small amounts because they cannot be manufactured from other foods nor from within the body. Omega-3 and omega-6 fats – the essential fatty acids – are crucial for normal growth and development.
∗ Cutting down on fatty foods is the fastest way to reduce your calorie intake but if you go too low you may

get bored and drive yourself into an eating frenzy!
∗ Fat acts as an important carrier for fat-soluble vitamins (A, D, E and K) in the bloodstream.
∗ Your liver produces cholesterol irrespective of the cholesterol in your diet.
∗ Cholesterol in food has less effect on your blood cholesterol than animal (saturated) fats.
∗ What you replace saturated fats with, as well as how much you eat, has been shown to be beneficial to overall health (see 'Get your fats straight').

if you replace saturated fat with sugar or low fibre carbs, this can increase your risk of heart disease. If the saturated fat is replaced by unsaturated fat (like olive oil), the risk appears to be reduced.

There are good research studies to suggest that a number of types of saturated fatty acids increase your blood cholesterol. However, one of the most common saturated fats in the diet (stearic acid, which you find in beef and dairy products) does not seem to have a negative effect on cholesterol. Because most fats and oils are made up of a mixture of different fatty acids, this area can get confusing. Just remember that all fats give you more than twice the calories of sugar or carbs, so cutting down on fatty and fried foods can help you keep to a healthy weight, which in turn can help reduce your risks of heart disease.

Get your fats straight
Fats differ according to their chemical make-up. Not all saturated fats are bad for you, but we do know that eating a lot of them is bad for your health. Most people in the UK eat too much saturated fat – the Department of Health's Food Standards Agency recommend that no more than 11 per cent of your daily calorie intake should come from this group. That equates to about a maximum of 30g per day for an average man, and 20g per day for an average woman. The rest of your fat intake should come from monounsaturated and polyunsaturated fats. Put simply:

✳ Too many saturated fats can raise blood cholesterol.

✳ Replace saturated fats with unsaturated fats to lower your risk of heart disease.

Fats	Examples	Recommendations
Monounsaturates	Olive oil, rapeseed oil groundnut oil, spreads made from these oils	There are good replacements for saturated fats
Omega-3 polyunsaturated fats	Fish oils, rapeseed oil, olive oil, spreads made from fish oils, linseeds, soya beans. Oily fish like mackerel, salmon, sardines and trout are a good source of omega-3 fats	Choose one portion of oily fish a week
Omega-6 polyunsaturated fats	Soya margarines, sunflower spreads, sunflower, soya bean, safflower, corn and grapeseed oils	Replace saturates with these, but eat in moderation
Trans fats	Hydrogenated spreads, processed foods made with trans fats	Keep to a minimum, remove from diet where possible
Saturates	Butter, lard, coconut oil, animal suet, processed foods made with saturates, fatty meat, skin	Keep to 30g limit for men and 20g limit for women
Cholesterol	Eggs, shellfish, offal	Eat in sensible amounts as part of an overall balanced eating plan

✳ Eating more plant-based foods is good for your health. Replace foods rich in saturated fats with whole grains, fish, pulses, vegetables and nuts.

✳ Trans fats are usually by-products of hydrogenation, a process used to make unsaturated fats firm and spreadable. Research has shown that they raise blood cholesterol. Trans fats are found in processed foods like biscuits, cakes and pastries (check the labels).

✳ Dietary cholesterol has little effect

on blood cholesterol. A low-fat diet will generally also be low in cholesterol, so you need not be overly conscious of cholesterol levels in food (unless you have a blood disorder, which specifically requires dietary cholesterol modification).

Reducing fat in cooking
Use cooking-oil sprays, which are often a mixture of oil and water (make your own using 1 part oil to 7 parts water, or use a drizzle of olive or rapeseed oil), or a small amount of butter in cooking. Try reduced-fat dairy products, such as semi-skimmed or skimmed milk, half-fat

dressings on low-fat natural yogurt and lemon juice, or buy fat-free dressings.

Should you switch to coconut oil, olive oil or butter?

There has been a lot of promotion of the value of coconut oil, both as a cosmetic and in nutrition, but what's the truth? Coconut oil is high in saturated fats, some of which are the ones known to increase cholesterol. So, from that point of view it's perhaps not ideal. Also, like all fats, it's extremely high in calories, meaning the claims that it can help weight loss do not really stack up. Add to this the cost, and it is certainly not the magic bullet many are looking for! On the plus side, some say they can get away with using less coconut oil than other fats so that might help; also it is a great alternative for lard in pastry, especially for vegetarians.

A lot of attention is given to olive oil, as it is rich in monounsaturated fats, which can both help to lower and improve balance of cholesterol. It has also been shown (when added to a Mediterranean type diet) to reduce incidence of heart disease. On the downside, it can 'smoke' if used to fry at high temperatures, so another mono-unsaturated oil, rapeseed oil, may be a better option for cooking.

For all fats, it's not a good idea to start eating more, and the same is true of butter. Using a little in cooking and spreading can increase flavour, but too much can increase your calorie intake and may raise your cholesterol.

The bottom line: use small amounts of the type of fat that works best in your recipe, but watch the total amount you eat in a day and bear in mind that deep frying is not a healthy choice.

Protein

The majority of people in the Western world eat more than enough protein and deficiency is extremely rare. Some people need more protein – if you're recovering from an illness, for example. People with diabetes may be at higher risk of developing kidney problems (nephropathy) and are therefore advised to keep to sensible amounts and avoid higher-than-average intakes. This is especially important if you also have high blood pressure, which could increase the potential for damage. If you already have kidney damage, you may be advised to limit protein intake more strictly and the specialist advice of a registered dietitian will be necessary.

Which protein foods to choose?

There are vegetable (e.g. beans, pulses, nuts) and animal (e.g. meat, dairy products) sources of protein. Other than in the case of lean meat, fish and low-fat dairy products, animal sources do tend to be higher in saturated fat. Studies have found lower blood cholesterol and blood pressure and better blood-sugar control in people with diabetes who follow predominantly plant protein-based diets rather than in those who follow animal-based ones.

Combined food group	Food examples	Recipe ideas
Cereals and pulses	Wheat and beans	Baked beans on toast Bruschetta with white bean purée and raw mushrooms (page 78)
	Rice and kidney beans	Jamaican rice and peas Vegetable chilli
	Rice or noodles and soya beans	Tofu stir-fry
	Wheat and lentils	Lentil soup and bread
	Rice and lentils	Dhal curry and rice
	Sweetcorn and beans	Tortilla and refried beans
Cereals and nuts	Wheat and peanuts	Peanut butter sandwich
	Wheat and nuts	Nut roast with breadcrumbs Chicory salad with walnuts and croûtons (page 65)
Pulses and seeds	Chickpeas and sesame seed paste	Hummus

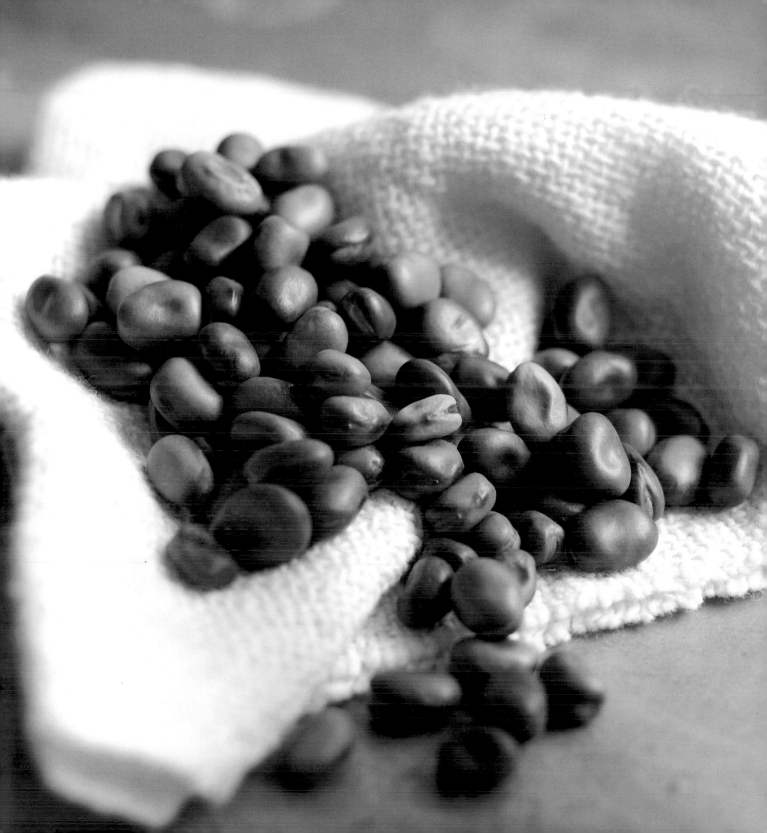

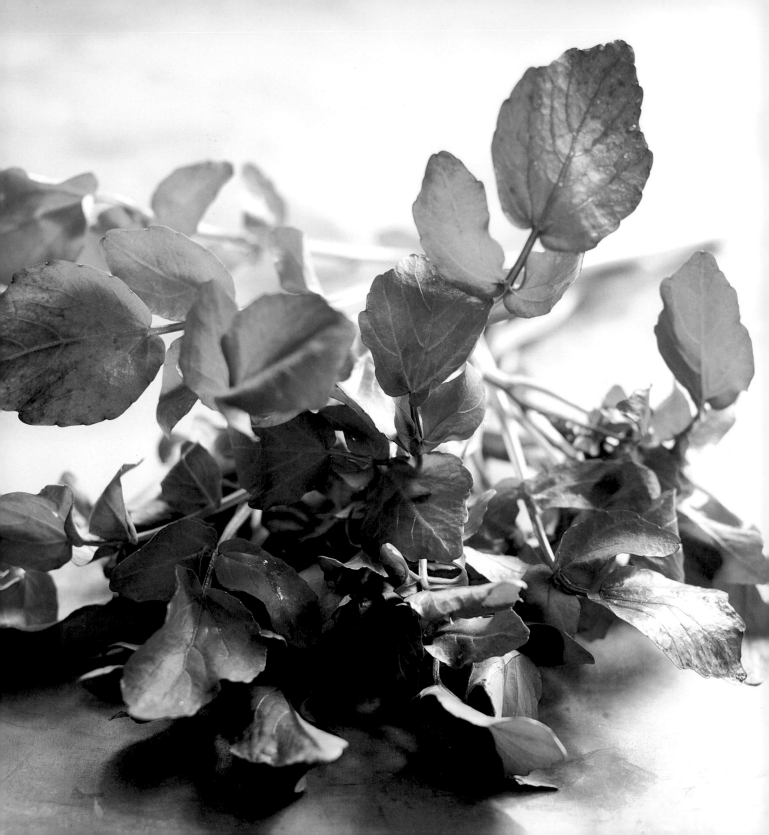

This doesn't mean you should become a vegetarian. Simply vary your meals so that you include a good range of vegetarian foods often.

All proteins are made up from building blocks called amino acids, some of which are essential to the body. Vegetable proteins tend to be lacking in one or more essential amino acids but if you mix them together, you can achieve the right balance. Many vegetarian dishes are based on this principle. The table on page 18 offers tips on how you might combine vegetable protein foods to get the best mix.

Fruit and vegetables

These foods contain important vitamins that are needed for health, whether you have diabetes or not. A diet that contains plenty of fruit and vegetables will provide more fibre and more vitamins, and will usually be lower in fat. The vitamins, beta-carotene (which is converted to vitamin A in the body), vitamins E and C, have been linked to a lower incidence of heart disease, some cancers and gut problems.

It is recommended that you eat at least five portions of fruit and vegetables daily. Try to do the following.
• Choose fruit and vegetables of varying colours – a wide range of colours will give you a wider variety of nutrients.
• Steam them quickly in the minimum amount of water in a covered pan – this helps to preserve the vitamin C.
• Serve them as whole as possible rather than puréed. Mashing or puréeing tends to raise the glycaemic index.

How much is enough?
For good health, you should aim for at least 400g, or about five 80g portions per day. Potatoes are classified as starchy carbohydrates, so they don't count.

What constitutes a portion?
∗ Medium apple, pear, orange, banana

∗ Large slice of melon or pineapple

∗ Cupful of strawberries or grapes

∗ 1 heaped tablespoon of dried fruit

∗ 2 small fruits, e.g. plums or satsumas

∗ 1 small glass (150ml) of fresh fruit juice

∗ 3 tablespoons of cooked vegetables

∗ Dessertbowl of salad vegetables, e.g. a carrot, a tomato, or a small bowl of mixed salad

∗ 3 tablespoons of tinned vegetable, e.g. sweetcorn, baked beans. Pulses, such as beans and lentils, can only be counted as one portion a day, as they don't contain the range of nutrients you get from other sources such as green leafy vegetables, carrots and tomatoes.

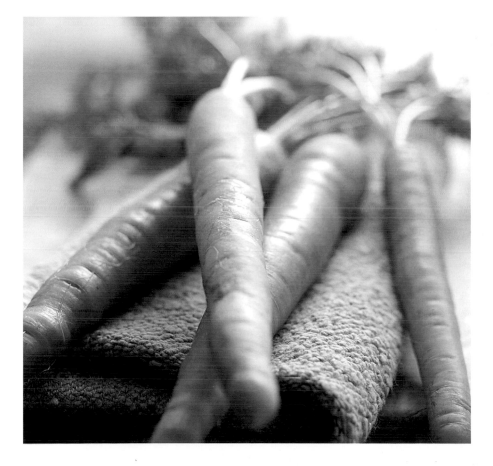

What about juice and smoothies?

As you can see from the list, fresh fruit juice does count, but choose 150ml of fruit juice only once a day, since the valuable fibre has been removed.

From the diabetes point of view, drinking large amounts of fruit juice, even if this is unsweetened, may make your blood glucose rise sharply. This is because the natural sugar in a liquid form is rapidly absorbed by the body. If you like fresh fruit juice, drink a 150ml glass with a meal rather than on its own. Alternatively, choose a sugar-free squash or diet drink.

Although fruit juice is a source of 'free sugars', it is a valuable provider of micronutrients like potassium, vitamin C and folate. When it comes to smoothies, the juice part is free sugars; the rest is pulped fruit. A 250ml serving of a smoothie counts as two of your five a day, so long as it contains 80g fruit and/or veg plus 150ml fruit juice. And since a serving of smoothie already has 150ml fruit juice in it, it's best you don't drink both smoothies and fruit juice on the same day.

Smoothies are made up of a mixture of fruits, so they give you a wider range of nutrients, and are also a source of fibre. Check the label for sugar content and watch your portion size.

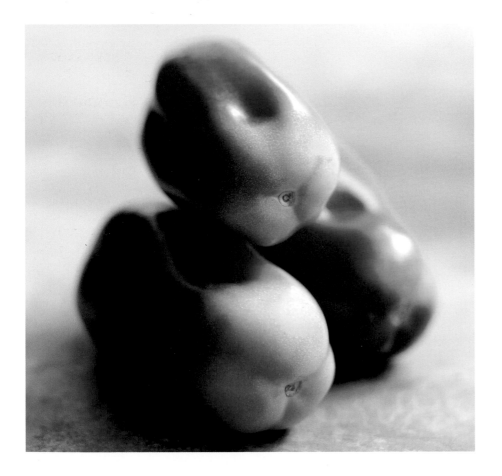

Meat, fish, nuts, pulses and eggs

These foods are rich in protein and many are good sources of vitamins and minerals, such as iron and zinc. However, fatty cuts of meat can be high in saturated fat, so it is best to choose lean cuts and to minimise the oil you use in cooking.

Meat dishes can be made healthier by adding beans or vegetables. This adds fibre, makes the meal go further and generally provides fewer calories per plate.

Salt and hypertension

High blood pressure makes you more prone to heart conditions, and eating too much salt is linked with high blood pressure and strokes. Salt is the common name for sodium chloride and it is the sodium part of salt which is harmful if taken in excess. It's estimated that people in the UK currently eat at least 10 grams or 2 teaspoons of salt each day. Most of the salt we eat comes from manufactured foods, and you may well be consuming far more than this amount each day, especially if you rely heavily on processed meals and snacks or takeway foods. For good health, it is recommended that you keep your total daily salt intake (including that in manufactured foods) to a maximum of 6 grams, or just over 1 teaspoon. This is equivalent to 2.5g of sodium.

Salt sense

✳ Measure the amount of salt you add in cooking and gradually cut down till a recipe that serves four people contains around ½ teaspoon of salt.

✳ Avoid adding salt at the table.

✳ Experiment with herbs and spices, using, for example, freshly ground spices, dried and fresh herbs, paprika and freshly milled black pepper. If you find it hard to get used to a less salty flavour, you can try a salt substitute. (Note that these are based on potassium chloride, so if you have a kidney disease these are best avoided). Reduced salt foods (such as vegetables canned in water, unsalted butter) can be used as replacements.

✳ For varied flavours, try lime juice, balsamic vinegar and chilli sauce.

✳ Read food labels carefully. Salt may appear as sodium, sodium chloride, monosodium glutamate or bicarbonate of soda. Multiply the sodium figure by 2.5 to find the salt content.

✳ Cut down on salty foods such as salted crisps, salted nuts, savoury biscuits and pastries.

✳ Processed and smoked foods such as bacon, sausages, smoked fish, some canned fish, etc., are often loaded with salt. Whenever possible, use fresh foods such as fish, lean meat, fruit and fresh vegetables. They have only a small amount of salt.

Salt substitutes

If you need to cut down on salt, you will find that in time your taste buds adjust and you will begin to prefer the taste of less salty foods. If you are still craving a salty flavour, however, a salt substitute is a practical and convenient way of reducing your salt intake. Read the label – some leading brands offer up to two thirds less sodium than ordinary salt, and you can use them in cooking and at the table. They are not recommended for people with kidney problems, however, as they contain potassium which can have a harmful effect on diseased kidneys.

Alcohol

If you have diabetes there's no reason why you shouldn't enjoy a drink, unless, of course, you have been advised to avoid alcohol for another medical reason.

Observe the safe drinking limit for everyone: the latest guidance is no more than 14 units each week for men or women, spread out over 3 days or more. Note that these are the maximum recommended amounts and drinking less is preferable. Try to space your drinking throughout the week and to have two or three alcohol-free days each week.

Safe drinking

Alcohol can cause hypoglycaemia (a 'hypo', or low blood glucose, see page 8) if you are taking insulin or certain tablets for your diabetes, and the higher the alcohol content (such as in spirits), the more likely it is to cause a hypo. Here are some guidelines which may help to prevent this:

✳ Avoid drinking on an empty stomach. Always have something to eat with a drink and especially afterwards if you have been out drinking. This is because the hypoglycaemic effect of alcohol can last for several hours.

✳ Choose low-alcohol drinks; avoid special diabetic beers or lagers, as these are higher in alcohol.

✳ If you enjoy spirits, try to use the sugar-free/slimline mixers.

✳ If you count the amount of carbohydrate you eat, don't include the carbs from alcoholic drinks.

✳ Drink less if you are trying to lose weight and consume no more than 7 units of alcohol per week.

Know your units

Pub measures seem to have increased over the years. The following guide can be found on the NHS Choices website, which also offers a calculator to help you monitor your drinking habits.

✳ Small glass wine (125ml): 1.5 units
✳ Standard glass wine (175ml): 2.1 units
✳ Large glass wine (250ml): 3 units
✳ Pint of lower strength beer: 2 units
✳ Pint of higher strength beer: 3 units
✳ Alcopop (275ml): 1.5 units
✳ Single shot of spirits (25ml): 1 unit

diabetes education

Living with diabetes is challenging. It can require large adaptations to lifestyle for the person living with the condition. To help with this, a lot of support and knowledge is needed to maximise quality of life and health. To support this, within the UK structured diabetes education has become a routine part of diabetes care. The purpose of this is to provide support and education to empower people with diabetes to be able to effectively self manage their condition. This has involved organised groups developing so that these programmes have a defined philosophy of education, a written and reproducible curriculum, trained educators and a system that reviews how effective the programmes are. There are separate education programmes for people with type 1 and type 2 diabetes, which are typically delivered to groups of 6–20 people. Working with groups allows people to share experience and learn about their conditions together with the healthcare professional having more of a supporting role.

The Dose Adjustment For Normal Eating programme (DAFNE) for Type 1 Diabetes

For people with type 1 diabetes, education programmes focus on estimating the amount of carbohydrate in foods and then working out doses of insulin to match to the food. Along with these principles of carbohydrate counting and insulin dose adjustment, aspects including eating out, effects of alcohol, illness and exercise are also discussed. The most widely used program in the UK (along with Australia and Ireland) is DAFNE (Dose Adjustment for Normal Eating). This is typically delivered as a 5-day course with follow-up sessions. These are full days supported by specialist nurses, dietitians and doctors, which are fully interactive building confidence in estimating carbohydrate content of foods, and looking for patterns in glucose readings to choose insulin doses. This approach was originally developed in Germany, in Dusseldorf, first being delivered in the UK in 1997. Since, then there has been an expansion across the UK with over 3,500 people attending last year. In addition there are many local courses based on the principles of dose adjustment of insulin and counting carbohydrate intake.

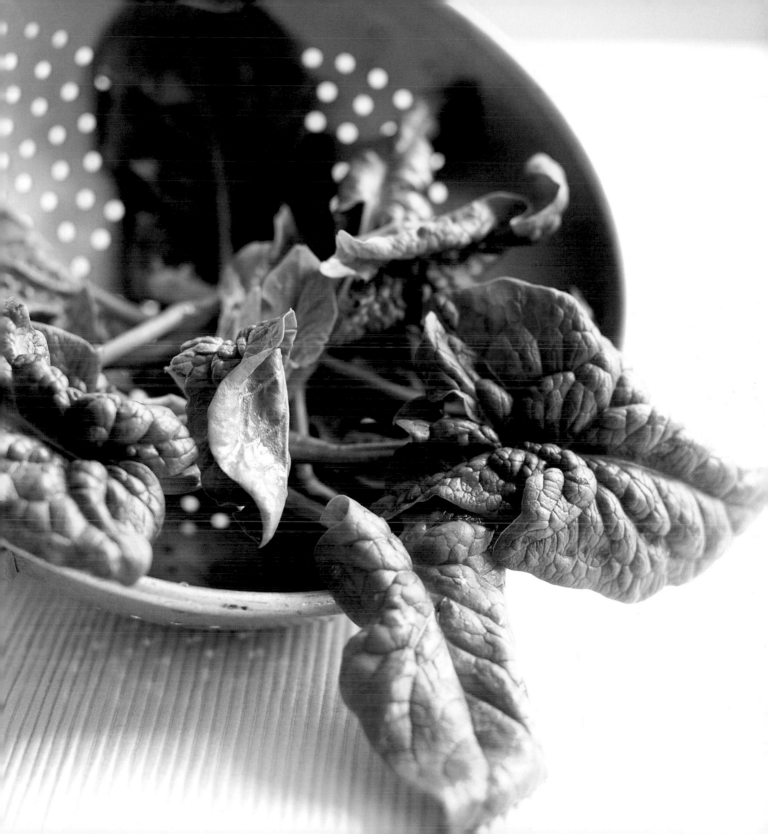

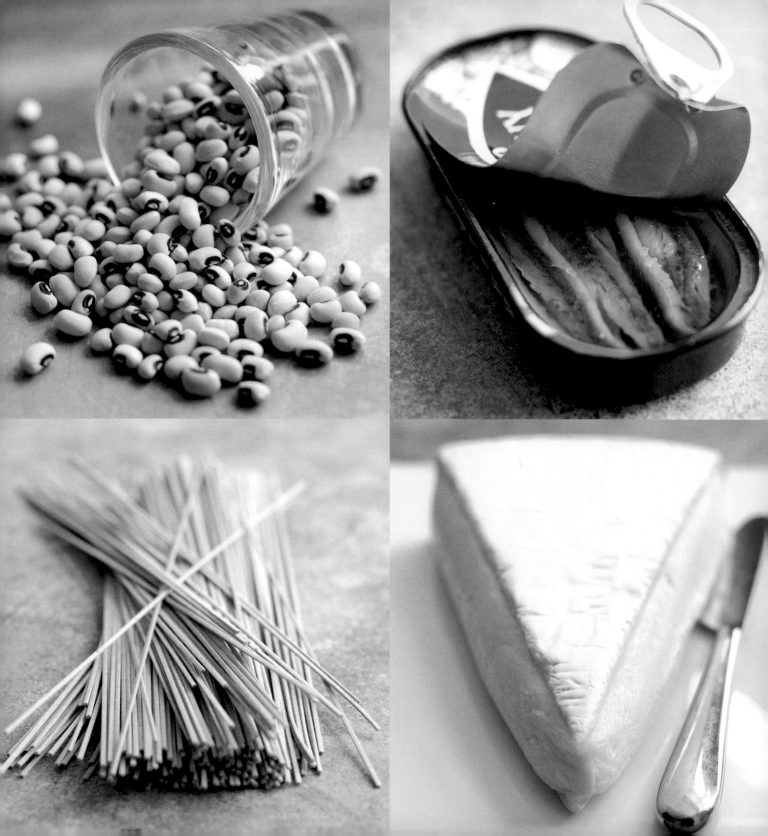

recipe tips for diabetes

All the recipes in this book are in line with healthy eating principles and they use lower fat, lower glycaemic index ingredients as appropriate. At times you will find that some dishes may appear to be 'no-go areas' for people with diabetes, but we want to dispel the myth that people with diabetes need a special diet. All your favourite foods can be incorporated into a healthy way of eating – it's getting the combinations right that's important and making sure that you choose a variety and watch your portion size.

Tempting desserts and main meals cooked in creamy sauces may sound off limits, but these recipes have been originated with diabetes in mind, using ingredients such as lean meat, fromage frais, half-fat crème fraîche, lower-fat Greek yogurt and skimmed milk. Asian-style dishes are served with steamed rice rather than fried rice, and in some recipes fat has been trimmed off meat after cooking, such as in Ham Bollito (page 120), so that the fat content will actually be lower than in the analysis given in the recipe.

Cooking tips

✳ Select lean cuts of meat and trim off visible fat. Try to cook meat without adding fat by grilling, roasting and braising. Avoid using the juices from roast meat for gravy.

✳ Remove the skin from poultry and remember that the thigh and leg pieces are highest in fat.

✳ Grill chops and burgers and allow the fat to drain off.

✳ If you need to fry foods, try a drizzle of oil or cooking-oil spray on a non-stick pan and stir-fry or sauté.

✳ Use whole-grain carbohydrate foods such as whole-grain bread and cereal, and brown pasta.

✳ Remember the Mediterranean 'musts' (see page 10) – fruit, vegetables, fish, nuts, beans, lentils.

✳ Select foods with a lower glycaemic index, (GI; see page 13). Foods that are high in soluble fibre, such as rye, granary and soft-grain white bread, peas, sweetcorn, beans, lentils, citrus fruits and porridge oats, typically have a low GI. Pulses such as beans, sweetcorn, peas and lentils are generally low in calories and help to fill you up.

✳ Include lots of fish and try to include oily fish such as salmon, herring and mackerel once a week.

✳ Nuts, although high in fat, can be part of a healthy lifestyle. Research shows that a handful of peanuts or almonds can help to lower your risks of heart disease. Nuts are best used as an ingredient in a main meal rather than as a snack, especially if you are overweight. Choose unsalted types.

Give these a miss...	... and try these instead!
Cheddar cheese	French Brie or low-fat soft cheese, or a smaller amount of grated extra mature Cheddar
Rich desserts	Fruity puddings
French fries or mashed potato	Whole new potatoes boiled in their skins
Fatty meat	Lean meat, poultry without the skin, fish
Flaky pastry	Filo pastry with skimmed milk between layers
Mayonnaise	Reduced-calorie mayonnaise or fat-free dressings
Full-fat dairy products, e.g. full-fat milk/cheese, butter	Reduced-fat foods, e.g. semi-skimmed milk, half-fat cheese, reduced- or low-fat spread
Cooking oil for frying	Spray oil for greasing and shallow-frying, a little olive or rapeseed oil for stir-frying, sautéeing, etc.
Crisps and salty snacks	Home-made popcorn, Melba toasts, pretzels, bread sticks, unsalted nuts
Rich cakes	Scones, fruit loaf, sponge cake

eating out

In today's hectic lifestyle, food on the go is becoming more and more common, and keeping an eye on the fats and figures can often become quite difficult as a result. What's more, fast food isn't necessarily healthy food, and often convenience overtakes health. So what are the best choices you can make to fit in with the chaos of modern-day life?

Going for an Indian

Opt for grilled chicken, prawn or vegetable dishes rather than rich curries, which tend to be higher in fat – tandoori chicken, with plain boiled rice and some cucumber raita is a good choice. Tikka dishes or a small portion of grilled kebabs make good starters. Opt for dhal (lentil) dishes instead of veggie curries, as they tend to be less oily. Pilau rice is fried rice, often with coloured grains – order boiled rice to keep the calories low. Basmati rice also has a lower GI than other types of rice, which is good news. Ask if your poppadam can be microwaved or grilled, and your chapatis or naan served dry.

Some restaurants refer to Indian cheese, paneer, as cottage cheese, but watch out as it's actually full-fat cheese.

The chippie

Thick-cut chips absorb less fat than thin-cut ones, as the thin ones have a larger surface area, but do watch out for those massive portion sizes at the local chippie.

Try bringing your chips home and sitting them on kitchen paper – if you want to microwave them, do so for a few seconds on the kitchen paper and see the fat soak in. You could take the batter off the fish, or if you want to be neat, place the fish, skin side down, on a plate. Use your fork and eat the top layer of batter with the fish only, leaving the skin side on the plate.

For a healthier option, go for grilled fish if available, bread roll and a salad accompaniment.

Burger binge

Burgers seem to be getting bigger as fast food chains bring out super-sized options. Top with a dressing and cheese and the calories start to soar. Pile on the fries and soft drink, and things really start to get out of hand. And the veggie-burger option is not necessarily any more virtuous. This is generally still cooked in fat and served with a creamy dressing.

Check out the calorie content on the menu board or nutrition leaflets – calorie values are now increasingly on show in large fast food outlets. This can be really helpful information if you're watching your weight. Order diet drinks and omit creamy dressings and sauces.

Here's a tip: munch through an apple or banana on your way to the burger bar, to take the edge off your appetite and help you resist the temptation to go super-sized.

Going Greek

Fill up on a starter of tzatziki – a low-fat mixture of yogurt, cucumber and garlic – with a small piece of pitta bread, instead. Go for Greek salad drizzled with fresh lime juice and smothered in coarsely ground black pepper. For your main, try grilled fish, grilled lean lamb chops or chicken skewers. A veggie option like falafel is usually deep-fried and therefore not necessarily lower in calories. Ask for fewer falafel balls and fill the pitta bread with some tzatziki and loads of salad.

Chinese food

A common pitfall when eating Chinese, Indian and Thai meals is ordering group dishes. This can often lead you to go for second or even third helpings! Try to give yourself a full plate at the beginning of a meal and stop when it's finished. Pile up the salad and vegetables as they help to fill you up.

Order plain boiled rice or noodles rather than the special fried varieties. Soft noodles with vegetables (such as a chow mein dish) are preferable to crispy ones. Go for steamed dishes, like a whole steamed fish with ginger, steamed vegetables and steamed rice. Choose healthy starters like satay dishes with chilli dipping sauce, and finish with fresh fruit or a scoop of ice cream rather than the fried fritters.

Pasta and pizza

Remember that pasta has a low GI (see page 13) as long as you don't have a massive portion. Ask for a fresh tomato sauce, which tends to be lower in fat than cream-based sauces, and say 'no' to extra Parmesan cheese. Go for a thin-based pizza with masses of vegetable toppings and steer clear of extra cheese, pepperoni and deep-pan dishes.

Vegetarian dining

It's often thought that vegetarian foods are healthier, but this is not always the case. Dishes that are based on eggs and cheese can be high in fat – Cheddar cheese, for example, has around 30 per cent fat, mostly saturated. And don't be fooled into thinking that all foods bought from a health-food shop are good for you. Many can be high in fat and sugar, and even though they may have been made with wholemeal flour, they are not necessarily healthy.

If you are vegetarian, pulse vegetables such as beans and lentils provide a valuable source of protein and have a low GI (see page 13). Use these together with wholegrain carbs like brown rice and pasta, and serve with lots of salad to prepare perfectly balanced meals (see the table on page 18).

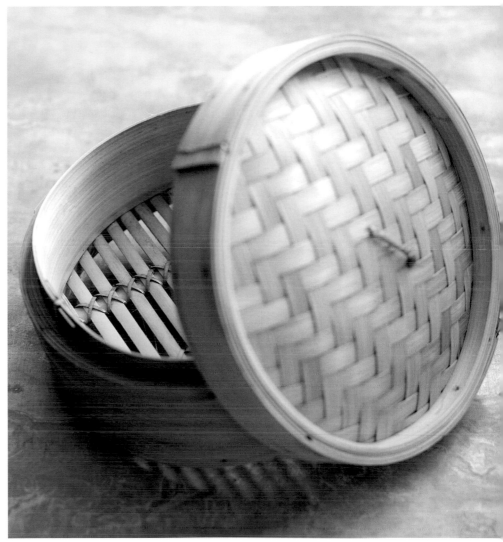

shopping

As we have seen so far, diabetes is about sensible and varied eating habits – not specialist health-food shopping. Imagine your supermarket trolley is divided into thirds. One third should be made up of fruit and vegetables; another could consist of bread, other cereals and potatoes. The rest of the trolley could contain equal amounts of meat and fish, milk and dairy food and even less fatty or sugary food. So try to spend more time looking at the variety of fruit and vegetables and wholegrain foods available and less time on fatty snack foods. This will help you to make healthier choices and will also add variety to your diet. Some people find that shopping on the Internet stops them from buying large packets of snack foods on special offer, and being away from the tempting smells of the in-store bakery can help, too.

What about convenience foods?

We are all tempted, at one time or another, by the myriad convenience foods on offer, be they ready meals, pasta sauces or desserts. Can they really be part of a healthy diet? Is it possible to mix and match to make them healthy?

Once again, it's all about balance and moderation. Many will be lower in fibre than home-made versions. If you find that this is the case, you can complement them with some extra grainy bread or a jacket potato. Another good tip is to get into the habit of serving them with extra vegetables or salad.

You may be concerned that quick or convenient foods may be high in fat, sugar and salt, all of which are relatively cheap ways for manufacturers to add flavour. But how can you tell? Sometimes it's easiest to look out for the 'healthy eating' logo used by all the major supermarkets, but you should take extra care with labels boasting 'healthy' on desserts and cakes, as they might be lower in fat but also higher in sugar, which does not necessarily mean that they are lower in calories.

Food labelling

Many foods make nutritional claims on their labels but research shows that consumers are very dubious as to how useful they really are. By law there are specific requirements a product must meet in order to make a nutritional or nutrient claim. Such claims may indicate a healthier choice, but bear in mind that this is all relative, as a reduced-fat version of a high-fat food could still be a high source of fat.

Understanding nutritional information on food labels

Whilst the ingredients list will tell you what's in a food, it does not tell you how much. Ingredients are listed in descending order of weight, so the first ingredient will be present in the largest quantity and the last ingredient will be the smallest. This can be useful up to a point but the actual nutritional content is

Guidelines to common nutrient claims (Food Standards Agency 2002)

Nutritional claim	Definition (per 100g or 100ml)	Example
Low sugar Low fat Low sodium	Contains less than 5g sugar Contains less than 3g fat Contains less than 40mg sodium	Sugar-free custard Low-fat rice pudding Low-salt foods
Reduced sugar Reduced fat Reduced salt	Contains 25 per cent less sugar, fat or salt than standard product	Reduced-sugar jams Reduced-fat spreads Reduced-salt baked beans
Sugar free	Contains less than 0.2g sugar	Sugar-free jellies Sugar-free squashes Sugar-free fizzy drinks (may be called 'diet')
No added sugar/ unsweetened	Contains no sugars or no added foods that are composed mainly of sugars	Unsweetened fruit juices

far more relevant. Even if sugar is near the top of the list, it does not necessarily mean that the food in question is packed with sugar. (Also remember that sugar does come in different guises, such as sucrose, dextrose, glucose syrup, maltose, etc.; see the table on page 12.)

Reference Intakes listed of food labels provide information on the average recommended nutrient content in a healthy diet for an adult of normal body weight. Exact needs will vary between individuals according to age, weight and physical activity level.

Nevertheless, RI can help you to see how and whether a particular food might fit into your diet.

Reference Intakes (RI) for adults

Nutrient	Average adult RI
Calories	2000
Fat	70g
Saturated fat	20g
Fibre	30g
Free sugars (not yet on label)	30g
Salt	6g

How do you compare foods?

Nutritional information can be used to tell you whether a food has a little or a lot of the listed nutrients. The table below provides guidelines to help you to determine this. When looking at food labels it is good practice to consider how often and in what amounts you would normally eat the food. A food may be high in fat and/or sugar, but if you eat only small amounts of it occasionally, that's acceptable.

For such foods you should refer to the 'per 100g' value; this is also useful for comparing two similar products such as ready-made sauces to see which is healthier. In the case of foods that you eat more frequently or in larger amounts, it is more appropriate to use the 'per serving' value.

Look out for red, green and amber traffic light labels on foods. These might make it easier for you to compare brands as you can opt for those that have fewer red lights.

NHS Choices guidelines on how to judge if a food is high or low in fat, sugar and salt

A lot/100g	A little/100g
More than 17.5g fat	3g fat or less
More than 5g saturates	1g saturates or less
More than 22.5g sugars	5g sugars or less
More than 0.5g sodium	0.1g sodium or less
More than 1.5g salt	0.3g salt or less

Healthy shopping tips

✳ Watch out for ever-increasing portion sizes on ready meals and snacks such as sandwiches, crisps and chocolate bars.

✳ Tinned foods such as fruit, vegetables, pulses and fish can be useful. Look for those labelled 'reduced' or 'no added' sugar or salt.

✳ Don't forget dried and frozen foods too – often just as nutritious and more convenient.

✳ Try to avoid shopping when you're hungry. Shop after a meal, make a shopping list and stick to it.

✳ Avoid foods such as biscuits and chocolates labelled 'suitable for diabetics'. They are usually expensive and have limited nutritional benefit. Since these are unlikely to form a major part of what you eat, you'd be better off just having a small amount of a standard product.

✳ Many supermarkets provide leaflets for people with diabetes, guiding them to healthy choices. Some even organise 'store tours' run by local registered dietitians. Consumers find these informative, enjoyable and a great way to view their regular store in a different light. Why not approach the customer services desk at your local store about this to generate demand?

watching your weight

Perhaps surprisingly, a heavy person burns more calories than a light person does, which destroys the myth that overweight people burn fewer calories when they exercise – often people who are overweight will blame their situation on a slow metabolism. It is possible to boost your metabolism by combining aerobic exercise and strength exercises.

Calories

The term 'calorie' is loosely used to describe the energy value of a food when the body burns it up. However, when talking about the measurement of energy, and hence how many calories a food has, the term kilocalories (or kcals) is more appropriate. On food labels, you will notice that the calorific value is given as kj/100g and kcal/100g. This means that every 100 grams of that product will provide you with the given amount of energy in kilojoules (kJ or kjoules) or kilocalories. One kcalorie is equivalent to 4.2 kjoules.

All the foods you eat provide calories, but some, generally those that are high in fat, are more concentrated in calories. For example, an apple, which is low in fat and high in fibre, will contain around 50 kcals, whereas an equivalent weight of Cheddar cheese will provide around eight times as many. Each gram of pure fat provides 9 kcals, whereas a gram of protein or a gram of carbohydrate will provide around 4 kcals. This is why frying a food can have a significant effect on the total calorie value.

Are you in shape?

Your ideal weight range depends on your height, and dietitians and doctors use each individual's body mass index (BMI) to calculate this. To find your BMI, take your weight (in kilograms) and divide it by your height (in metres squared):

$$BMI = \frac{weight\ (kg)}{height\ (m)^2}$$

The most desirable range is a BMI of between 20 and 24. A larger BMI is taken as an indication of being overweight and the higher that figure is, the more overweight you are.

The 'fruit salad' theory
Are you an 'apple', that is someone whose waist is bigger than their hips, or a 'pear', someone whose hips are bigger than their waist?

This may sound unimportant, but in fact real scientific theories have been formulated using this information. Central obesity, or putting weight on around the abdomen, is said to be associated with resistance to insulin, which in turn has been shown to be a risk factor in coronary heart disease (see metabolic syndrome, page 9). People with a higher waist measurement have a raised risk of diabetes and heart disease. A waist measurement of more than 94cm for men and more than 82cm in women is considered to carry a risk. Men of South Asian origin have been found to be even more at risk, so ideal waist measurements in their case need to be less than 92cm.

It would therefore appear that being more pear-shaped may actually offer some protection. Eating well and taking regular physical activity can help to reduce excess abdominal fat.

Steps to success

Before you begin your new healthy lifestyle, make a list of all the positive benefits you feel it will give you. Your list may include things like helping you to fit into those old jeans, being able to run for the bus (and catch it!), looking and feeling more confident, feeling less breathless, getting your blood cholesterol down so you don't need tablets, and so on. Think about what this new lifestyle, physique, and so on, will do for you. How will a new image affect other areas of your life – your confidence, your work performance, your social life, your belief in yourself? And how will it affect the way in which you interact with others – family, friends and colleagues?

If you are absolutely clear about why you would like a healthier lifestyle, you will vastly increase your motivation and therefore your chances of success.

A practical approach

Follow the nutritional guidelines in this book to help you achieve a balanced intake of the right types of foods. Start by making a note of exactly what you're eating (a food diary), so that you have a written record of days when perhaps things could have gone better. If you couple this with notes about how you were feeling at that particular time, a connection may begin to emerge between your moods and the times when you indulge. This can be useful in helping you to make lasting changes.

There's no need to cook separately for yourself. The best part about eating the right foods for slimming is that they're also great foods for the whole family. Simply serve yourself smaller portions and fill up on the vegetables and starchy foods. Don't skip meals, as this often makes you ravenous by the next meal and you're more likely to overdo it, or to snack on high-calorie foods in between. A healthy diet, tailored to your own individual needs may not sound as revolutionary as some of the 'miracle' diets endorsed by celebrities, but the evidence shows that it is the best way of losing weight sensibly and keeping it off. Registered dietitians can assess your current eating habits and lifestyle and advise you on appropriate strategies to lose weight slowly but steadily.

Think slim

✳ Often, keeping to a food plan means that you focus so much on food that you forget about the benefits of physical activity. Find ways of making exercise a part of your daily life in order to lose weight more quickly. Go for a brisk walk with a friend, splash around in the swimming pool or work out at the gym. Or, if you find it hard to make time for exercise, try running up and down the stairs at work a few times a day; or at

home, jog on the spot whilst watching your favourite soap.

✳ If you find yourself battling with food cravings, you have two choices: either eat a small amount, enjoy it and move on, getting quickly back on track. Or, think about how much slimmer and fitter you will be if you keep going, and decide that you won't be defeated by a chunk of cake which would probably disappear in seconds and be nothing more than a 'quick fix'.

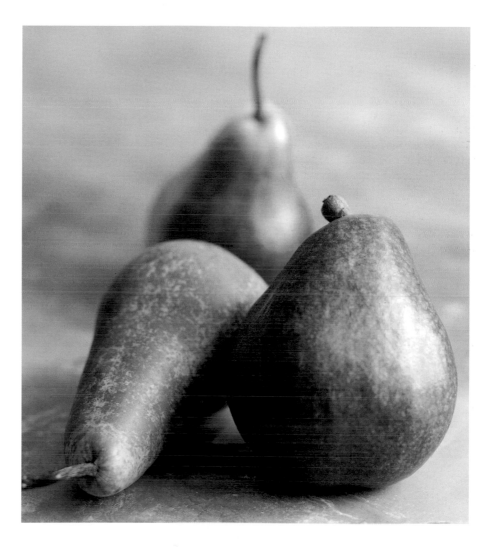

* Keep a 'thoughts' diary. Write down what you eat, when you eat it and what you were thinking at the time. You might find that the foods you would ideally like to eat less of creep into the menu when you're feeling low, fed up or bored. An awareness that you fall into this trap at certain times can help you to stay on track by planning ahead. When you feel down, do other things besides eating to pick yourself up – go for a stroll, listen to some music, phone someone for a chat, soak in the bath, read a magazine – anything that you enjoy that will give you more positive thoughts.

* Keep an eye on your eating habits. What time do you eat? Do you eat when you're hungry, or because, for example, it's mid-morning and everyone else is munching something? Are you a night-time snacker? If so, you could look at other ways of occupying yourself in the evenings to distract you from food. And if you must eat at night, choose healthier options, such as fruit, crudités with low-fat dips, fromage frais, diet yogurts, two crackers with a sliver of Cheddar cheese, a couple of Jaffa cakes or a handful of homemade popcorn. Eat from a smaller plate to make your meals look bigger.

* List all of the benefits that you hope to enjoy when you are fitter and healthier (see page 32). If you catch yourself straying, simply refer to your list and remind yourself of what you could achieve. Keep your list by the fridge, or anywhere eye-catching to keep you motivated.

Get physical

Physical activity helps your body to release endorphins, natural painkillers, which can in turn help you to combat stress and feel more energised. You don't need to jog ten times around the park or go to the gym every day in order to stay fit. Just try to incorporate simple activities into your daily lifestyle and gradually try to work up to 30 minutes a day, five times a week.

* Walk to the pillar box, take the dog out more often, take the kids for a brisk walk or simply park the car a bit farther away from your destination. Try to walk at a pace that leaves you slightly out of breath.

* Use the stairs instead of the lift whenever possible, or run up and down the steps at home a few times a day.

* Try skipping or jogging on the spot whilst watching TV.

* Take up a sport that you enjoy and which fits into your routine. Swimming with the kids or line dancing classes with a friend can be a fun way of working out.

* Remember that activity can be therapeutic, so tackling those garden weeds can have more benefits than you think.

And if you feel like giving it all up, take a look at your list of how great you'll feel when you get there and simply start again. You're human – it's perfectly acceptable to have 'off' days.

Keeping healthy – for life

In June 2002 the Diabetes Research and Wellness Foundation launched 'Think Well to be Well', a new concept in caring for people with diabetes. Bringing a fresh approach to diet and diabetes, the concept helps people with diabetes to take control of their life and to focus on achieving sustainable results. Let's take a look now at some practical steps based on this concept, which will allow you to challenge your thinking, helping you to achieve more long-term results.

Old habits die hard...
...so they say. But it's actually making that decision to make the change that takes longer. So start today by changing your attitude and you'll soon find other things changing with it.

What should you say to yourself?
The way you think can have a dramatic effect on your behaviour, including what you eat. The instructions that you feed your mind are what the mind will respond to. Practise giving yourself positive reinforcement and encouragement. Link these thoughts directly with your goal. For example, say things like, 'I feel better about myself when I eat fruit after lunch', or 'I'm doing well by walking more'. Imagine what others might say to support you, that would give you a positive feeling.

Your mind is programmed to give you more of whatever you are thinking about, so if you're thinking about being fat or unfit you are inadvertently programming yourself to get what you don't want. Tennis players, for example, know that if they worry about hitting the ball into the net, that is exactly where it is likely to go, so they focus on getting the ball just where they want it to go. The trick is to make conscious choices that bring you closer to your goal, in this case achieving a healthy lifestyle.

Keeping your diabetes in check

✳ Quit smoking now.

✳ Keep to recommended foods most of the time. The more low-GI (see page 13), balanced foods you eat, the better. Choose foods you enjoy and which fit in with your lifestyle, so that any changes are sustainable.

✳ Make sure you incorporate regular physical activity into your daily habits. This could be as simple as walking up the stairs, or parking the car a little farther away from your destination than normal.

✳ Keep to your prescribed dose of medication, unless it has been recommended by your medical advisers that you make changes.

✳ Check your blood glucose regularly so you can assess how your diabetes is at any given time.

✳ Attend your clinic for regular check-ups, and make sure that you monitor the health of your feet and eyes.

✳ Take appropriate action during periods of illness, or when going on holiday.

✳ Keep to within the maximum daily limits of alcohol (see page 23).

✳ Find ways of relaxing that will help you to combat stress.

Keeping the weight off
So you've done well and reached your desired weight. The last thing you want to do now is to put all that weight back on. But the sad fact is that most people who lose weight do regain it. So how can you make sure that doesn't happen to you? If your weight-reducing diet is something that you simply put up with until you reach your goal, then maybe it's the wrong diet for you. Seeing it as an endurance test is likely to make you indulge when it's over, which tends to make you fall back into those old habits. And then, of course, the weight creeps back on again.

Here are some 'think slim' tips:
✳ Treat your slimming plan as a new way of life. You may lapse occasionally – that's fine. Just acknowledge it and start again.

✳ Try to keep a sense of perspective about your weight – if you put on a pound or two, you can always take it off again.

✳ Challenge yourself. Now you have reached your target, what are you going to do next? Why not learn a new sport, or take up a new hobby?

✳ Find ways to make your work routine and your family support you. You are going to stay slim and healthy.

✳ Turn out your wardrobe and enjoy giving away clothes that are too big for you. Indulge yourself and buy some new clothes. If you make an effort to look good, you'll want to stay slim.

✳ Encourage your family and friends to join in with your exercise regime. It's much more fun to go cycling or swimming or play sport with other people.

✳ Keep a daily 'food and mood' diary so you can see when you indulge and what your emotions are up to at that time, e.g. boredom, stress, comfort, security, PMT.

✳ Before you reach for solace in that 'unhealthy nibble', ask yourself if choosing this is taking you nearer to the 'new' you, and if it isn't, choose again!

✳ Distract yourself. Perhaps make a creative list of all the things that would work for you, from going for a walk to having a bath or dancing to your favourite CD. By the time you've done this, your brain would have been sufficiently tricked into believing that it no longer needs that 'fix'!

from the chef

In 2003, I agreed to appear in a TV programme about sugar that involved having a test for metabolic syndrome (see page 9). I must have been mad – the things you do for telly! – but I knew a test this thorough was not available on the National Health Service. It was a complicated drawn-out test where glucose and insulin was pumped into my left arm and my right arm was placed in an 'oven' at 65°C (149°F). Blood was taken from it every 10 minutes for two hours and was then spun centrifugally to test my insulin resistance.

Shock, horror – I had metabolic syndrome; I was on my way to type 2 diabetes unless, that is, I took steps to change my lifestyle. With metabolic syndrome there is a way back, however, unlike with type 2.

It is estimated that between 20 and 25 per cent of the UK population has metabolic syndrome and they won't know a thing about it until it moves on to type 2 diabetes, and that will happen unless you take the right steps. Have a close look at your diet, take aerobic exercise to increase your heart rate for at least 20 minutes, four times a week, lose some of those pounds of flesh that seem to have come from nowhere and if you smoke, stop.

I have changed my lifestyle and hopefully I won't move on to the diabetes stage, but if I do then I'm determined still to enjoy my food. Wholesale changes aren't necessary; you can still eat normally and with the knowledge and advice we have given in this book, you will see life needn't change that much.

Although I wrote this book for people with diabetes, there is no harm in everyone getting stuck in too. Many of us need to watch what we eat, so there is no reason why you shouldn't have a lifestyle change straight away; an AWT meal a day may well keep metabolic syndrome away.

I'll be honest: out of choice I wouldn't use artificial sweeteners that contain aspartame, but natural substitutes for sugar are slowly finding their way on to the market. Even with metabolic syndrome I prefer not to use margarines or spreads containing trans fats or hydrogenated vegetable oils as there is more and more evidence that these can harm your health, but there are recipes in this book where there is no substitute. And I won't encourage you to drink artificially sweetened colas for the same reason, as you should try to discover more natural drinks. You can help yourself without reverting to science; natural foods unenhanced with chemicals are always going to be a better choice.

None of my recipes requires rocket science. Here are simple 'normal' recipes using a little knowledge and a lot of imagination to keep you enjoying your food. There is no regime, just common sense; no sergeant major barking orders, just foodie pleasure. Azmina has already explained the best balance of foods to eat. Remember that where a dish is to be served as a main meal you should ensure you serve it with extra vegetables or salad and some starchy carbohydrate when there is little or none in the recipe. Follow Azmina's advice and you'll soon realise that being diagnosed with diabetes need not be a trial or a long-term foodie prison sentence. Life is for living so give yourself that chance.

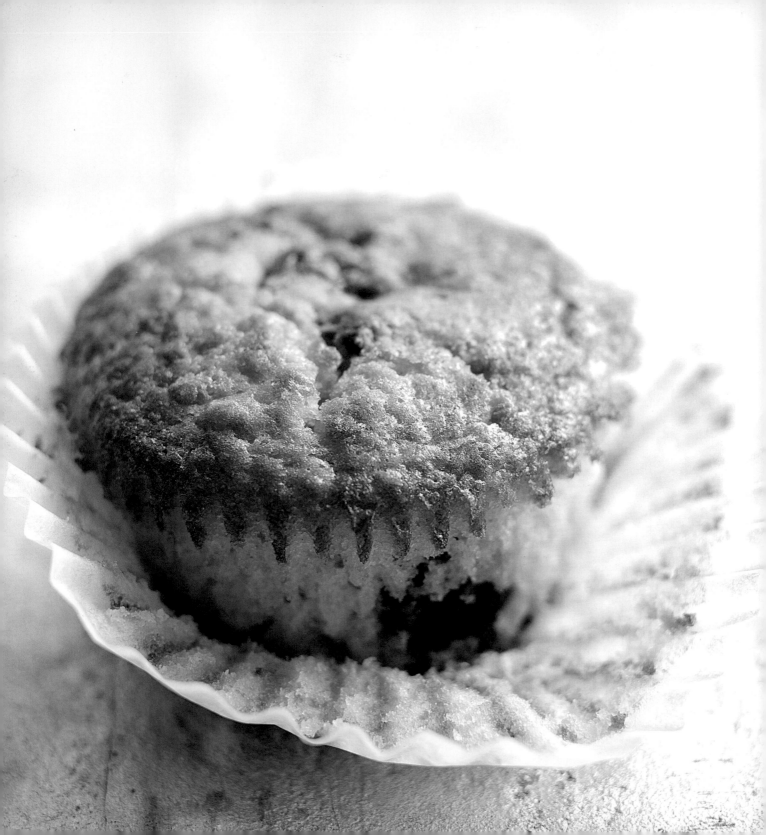

1

breakfasts
and brunches

asparagus, smoked bacon and spring onion hash

Perfect for a late brunch or lazy lunch, this classic dish combines great flavours with great textures.

1 garlic clove, finely chopped
2 spring onions, sliced into 2.5cm pieces
50g lean smoked bacon, diced
½ tablespoon rapeseed oil
1 teaspoon capers, drained and rinsed
8 cooked asparagus spears, cut into 5cm pieces
1 tablespoon black olives, pitted and diced
1 tablespoon balsamic vinegar
3 eggs
Freshly ground black pepper

Serves 2

In a non-stick pan, fry the garlic, spring onions and bacon in the oil until golden. Add the capers, asparagus, olives and vinegar and heat through.

Whisk the eggs and pour into the asparagus mix. Stir until the eggs are cooked to your liking and take on a scrambled appearance. Season with black pepper to taste and serve on granary toast.

PER SERVING:
203 KCALS, 14G FAT, 4G SATURATED FAT, 3G CARBOHYDRATE, 0.83G SODIUM

salmon and kipper kedgeree

A pleasant alternative to the usual smoked haddock version. Traditionally a recipe served at breakfast, this also makes a great light lunch, but eat once a week or so, rather than everyday.

1 kipper fillet
175g salmon fillet
1 bay leaf
150g brown rice
½ onion, chopped
25g unsalted butter
2 teaspoons curry paste
2 eggs, hard-boiled and chopped
2 tablespoons chopped parsley
Freshly ground black pepper

Serves 2

Cook the kipper and salmon in 600ml water with the bay leaf over a medium heat for 7 minutes, then allow to cool slightly. Discard the bay leaf and lift the fish out of the water, reserving the water. Flake the fish, discarding any skin or bone.

Rinse the rice, then measure 1 cup rice to 3 cups reserved fish cooking water into a pan, bring to the boil, reduce the heat and simmer covered, for about 30 minutes. Drain, separate the grains with a fork and set aside.

Meanwhile, cook the onion slowly in the butter until soft but not browned, add the curry paste and stir to combine. Add the rice, flaked fish, hard-boiled eggs and parsley and stir. Season with black pepper to taste and serve immediately.

PER SERVING:
766 KCALS, 40G FAT, 12G SATURATED FAT, 64G CARBOHYDRATE, 0.73G SODIUM

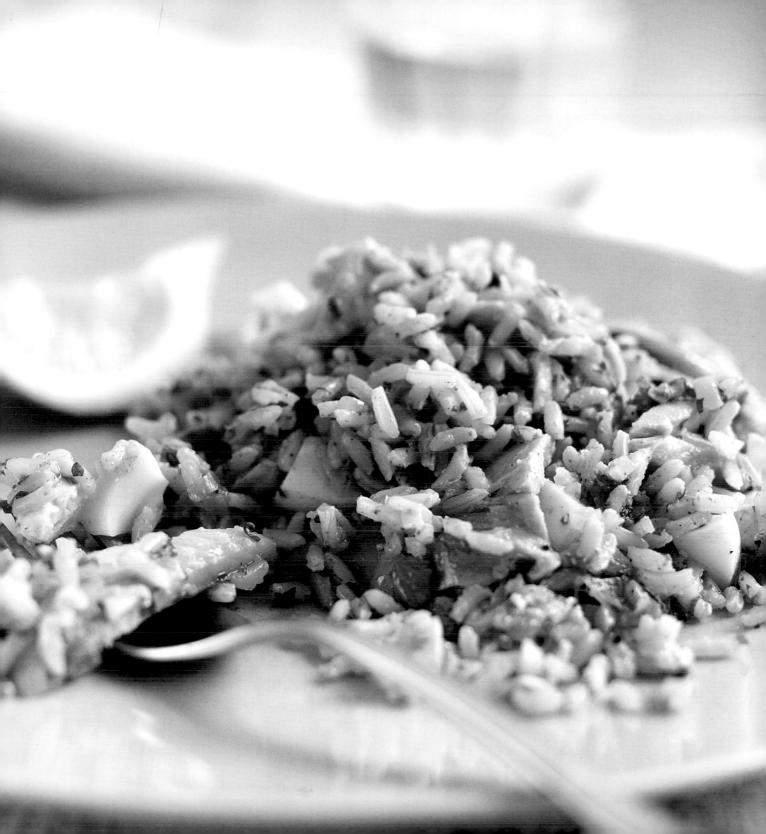

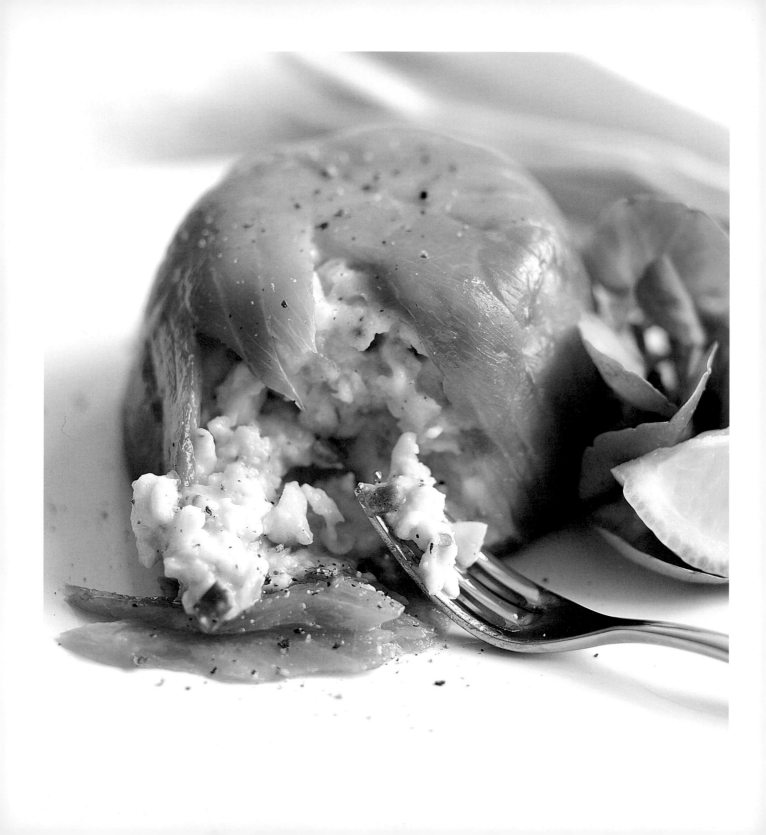

scrambled eggs and smoked salmon timbales

A classic dish, but given a more chef-style presentation. Two ingredients that combine to make the perfect breakfast. Serve with a slice of wholemeal toast.

Rapeseed-oil spray (see page 17)
110g smoked salmon, thinly sliced
4 eggs
2 teaspoons horseradish sauce
2 teaspoons snipped chives
Freshly ground black pepper
10g unsalted butter
Watercress, to garnish
Lemon wedges, to garnish

Serves 2

Lightly spray 4 timbales with oil and line with clingfilm.

Line each timbale with strips of smoked salmon, making sure there are no gaps and leaving an overhang to create a lid once the timbales are filled with scrambled eggs.

Lightly beat the eggs, folding in the horseradish and chives, but keeping some viscosity (in other words, don't overbeat). Season with pepper.

Melt the butter in a non-stick frying pan or saucepan until it foams, then pour in the eggs. With a wooden spoon, draw the edges of the eggs into the centre continuously until they have cooked to your liking. Immediately spoon the scrambled eggs into the smoked salmon moulds, push the eggs down with a teaspoon, then fold over the smoked salmon to enclose.

Turn the moulds out into the centre of 2 plates and garnish with any excess smoked salmon, the watercress and lemon wedges.

PER SERVING:
277 KCALS, 18G FAT, 6G SATURATED FAT, 2G CARBOHYDRATE, 1.22G SODIUM

baked egg in herbed roast beefsteak tomato

Eggs with inspiration. A wonderfully rich and filling dish, and the dash of Martini gives it a touch of decadence. Delicious with a slice of crusty bread.

50g button mushrooms,
  finely chopped
1 small onion, finely chopped
½ teaspoon soft thyme leaves
½ teaspoon ground black pepper
1 tablespoon olive oil
1 tablespoon dry Martini
4 beefsteak tomatoes

5 eggs
2 tablespoons low-fat
  Greek yogurt
2 teaspoons snipped chives
2 teaspoons finely chopped
  flat leaf parsley
Freshly ground black pepper

Serves 4

In a saucepan, cook the mushrooms, onion, thyme and black pepper in the olive oil on a gentle heat for about 15 minutes, stirring regularly until the onions have softened and the vegetables have released most of their liquid. Add the Martini and boil until all the liquid has evaporated, then set aside to keep warm. Preheat the oven to 180°C/350°F/gas mark 4.

Cut 1cm from the rounded end of each tomato. Hollow out the seeds and discard. Place the tomatoes cut side up on a roasting tray and cook for 10 minutes in the oven, with the lids placed separately on the roasting tray.

Meanwhile, beat one of the eggs. Whisk together the yogurt, herbs, 1 tablespoon water and the beaten egg. Remove the tomatoes from the oven and place a quarter of the mushroom mix in the bottom of each hollowed-out tomato. Break a raw egg on to the mushroom mix, spoon the yogurt mix over the egg and top each tomato with a tomato lid.

Return to the oven and cook for 10–15 minutes depending on how well you like your eggs cooked.

PER SERVING:
161 KCALS, 11G FAT, 3G SATURATED FAT, 6G CARBOHYDRATE, 0.11G SODIUM

scrambled crab

Eggs and crab make an excellent partnership and a more unusual combination than scrambled eggs and salmon. White meat comes from the claw of the crab and is the tastiest.

4 eggs
100g white crab meat
Freshly ground black pepper
2 slices wholegrain bread
10g unsalted butter
2 tablespoons low-fat Greek yogurt

Serves 2

Lightly beat the eggs, then combine with the crab meat. Season with ground black pepper. Toast the bread and spread with half of the butter. Keep warm.

Heat the remaining butter in a non-stick frying pan, pour in the eggs and stir until cooked to how you like your eggs. Fold in the yogurt and spoon on to the buttered toast.

PER SERVING:
337 KCALS, 19G FAT, 7G IS SATURATED FAT, 15G CARBOHYDRATE, 0.55G SODIUM

brown soda bread

This is the easiest bread in the world to make. An Irish speciality, it is raised with bicarbonate of soda and an acid, the soured milk or buttermilk, instead of yeast.

450ml semi-skimmed milk or buttermilk
Juice of 1 lemon (if using milk)
280g plain white flour
1 rounded teaspoon salt (optional)
1 rounded teaspoon bicarbonate of soda
280g stone-ground wholemeal flour

Makes 1 loaf

Preheat the oven to 230°C/450°F/gas mark 8.

To sour the milk, pour it into a large jug with the lemon juice. Allow to stand for 15 minutes to thicken before stirring. If you prefer, you can use buttermilk instead of souring the milk yourself.

Sift the white flour, salt (if using) and bicarbonate of soda, add the wholemeal flour, stirring to combine in a large bowl. Make a well in the centre and add the soured milk or buttermilk, little by little.

Working from the centre, combine the mixture either by hand or with a wooden spoon, adding more soured milk if necessary. The dough should be soft, but not sticky. If it becomes too wet, add more flour.

Turn out on to a floured board and knead lightly, just enough to shape into a round. Flatten slightly to about 5cm thick and place on a baking tray.

Using a floured large knife, mark a deep cross on top and bake in the oven for 15–20 minutes, then reduce the heat to 200°C/400°F/gas mark 6 for 20–25 minutes, or until the bread is cooked and the bottom sounds hollow when tapped.

PER QUARTER LOAF:
508 KCALS, 4G FAT, 2G SATURATED FAT, 105G CARBOHYDRATE, 0.75G SODIUM

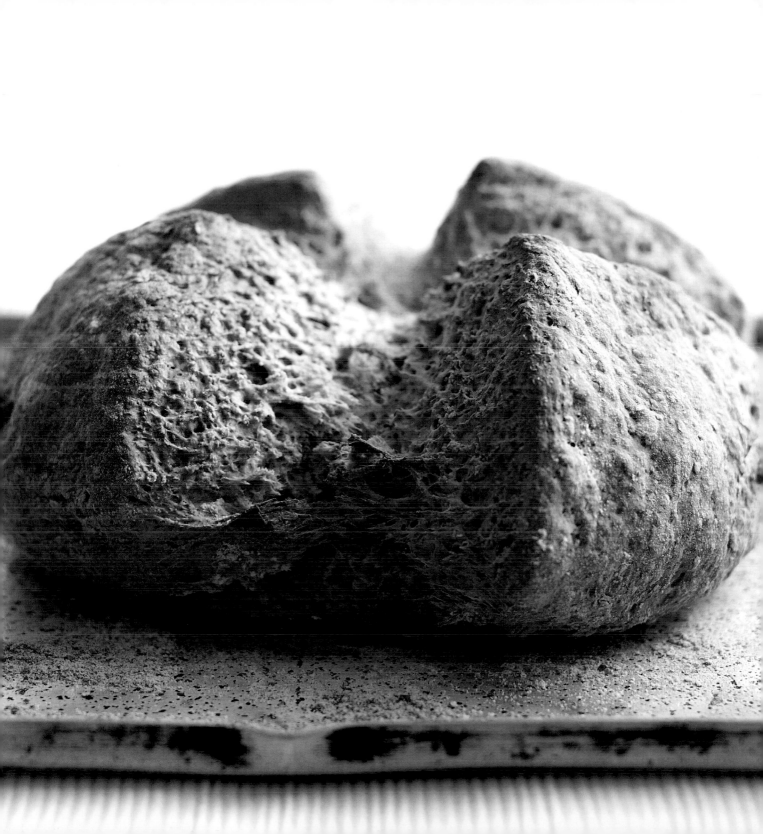

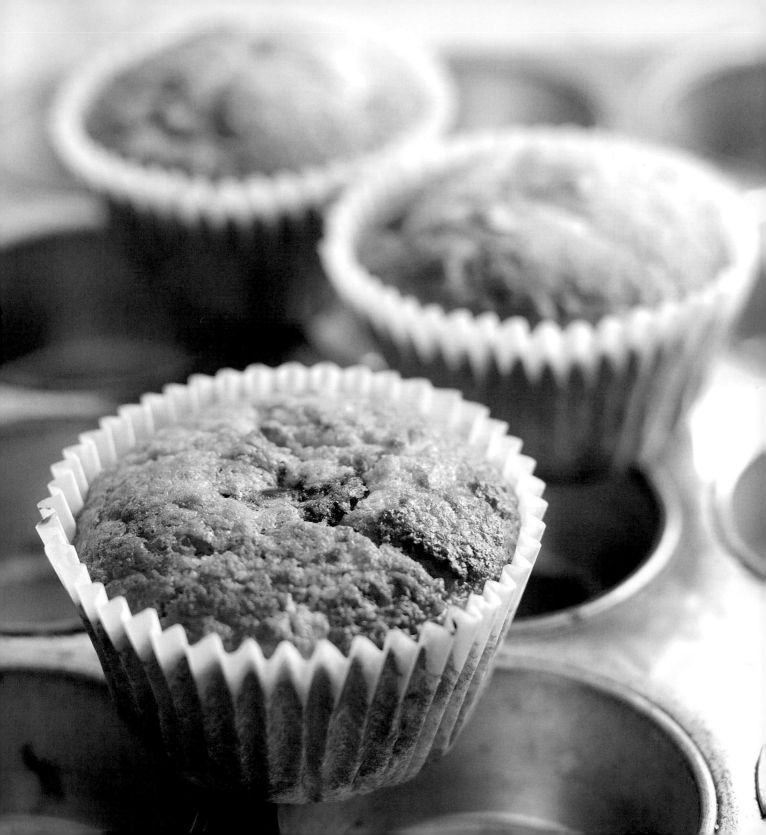

dried cherry muffins

Other dried fruit can be substituted, but I think that cherries are the most delicious. These muffins are great for a quick breakfast or mid-morning snack.

150ml semi-skimmed milk or buttermilk
1 tablespoon lemon juice (if using milk)
75g dried pitted cherries
150g plain flour

1½ teaspoons baking powder
50g unsalted butter
75g caster sugar
1 egg
½ teaspoon grated orange zest

Makes 12 small muffins

Preheat the oven to 180°C/350°F/gas mark 4.

If using milk, combine it with the lemon juice and leave to stand for 30 minutes.

If you have time, soak the cherries in the milk mix or buttermilk for 30 minutes. I know it's breaking the rules and isn't essential, but it does help to soften the cherries.

In a large bowl, sift together the flour and baking powder.

In a separate bowl, cream together the butter and sugar until light and fluffy. Lightly beat the egg, then add to the creamed butter together with the orange zest and combine. Make a well in the centre of the flour and baking powder and spoon in the cherries and soured milk or buttermilk. Add the butter mixture and mix the whole together with your hands until just combined. Don't overwork the batter.

Heap the mixture into the muffin cups, filling them two-thirds full. Bake in the oven for about 20 minutes, or until a skewer or cocktail stick inserted into the centre comes out clean. Transfer the muffins to a wire rack to cool.

PER MUFFIN:
131 KCALS, 5G FAT, 3G SATURATED FAT, 22G CARBOHYDRATE, 0.09G SODIUM

honey, orange and thyme bran muffins

There is plenty of fibre, but very little fat in these delicious muffins. Wheatbran is available from good health-food shops.

150ml semi-skimmed milk or buttermilk
1 tablespoon lemon juice (if using milk)
Rapeseed-oil spray (see page 17)
4 teaspoons soft light brown sugar
25g unsalted butter, melted

2 eggs, lightly beaten
½ teaspoon soft thyme leaves
60ml liquid honey
Grated zest of 2 oranges
110g plain flour
110g unprocessed wheat bran
3 teaspoons baking powder
Pinch of salt

Makes 12 muffins

Preheat the oven to 180°C/350°F/gas mark 4.

If using the milk, combine it with the lemon juice and leave to stand for 30 minutes.

Place the sugar in a bowl and combine with the melted butter, soured milk or buttermilk, eggs, thyme, honey and orange zest.

In another bowl, combine the flour, bran, baking powder and salt. Make a well in the dry ingredients and then fold in the milk mix. Combine until just mixed, but don't overwork the batter.

Fill each muffin cup two-thirds full with the batter and bake for 20–25 minutes until golden and cooked through. To test, insert a skewer into the centre of a muffin: if it comes out clean, the muffin is cooked. Remove from the oven, allow to stand for 10 minutes then turn the muffins out on to a wire rack to cool completely.

PER MUFFIN:
123 KCALS, 3.8G FAT, 1.6G SATURATED FAT, 19.6G CARBOHYDRATE, 0.22G SODIUM

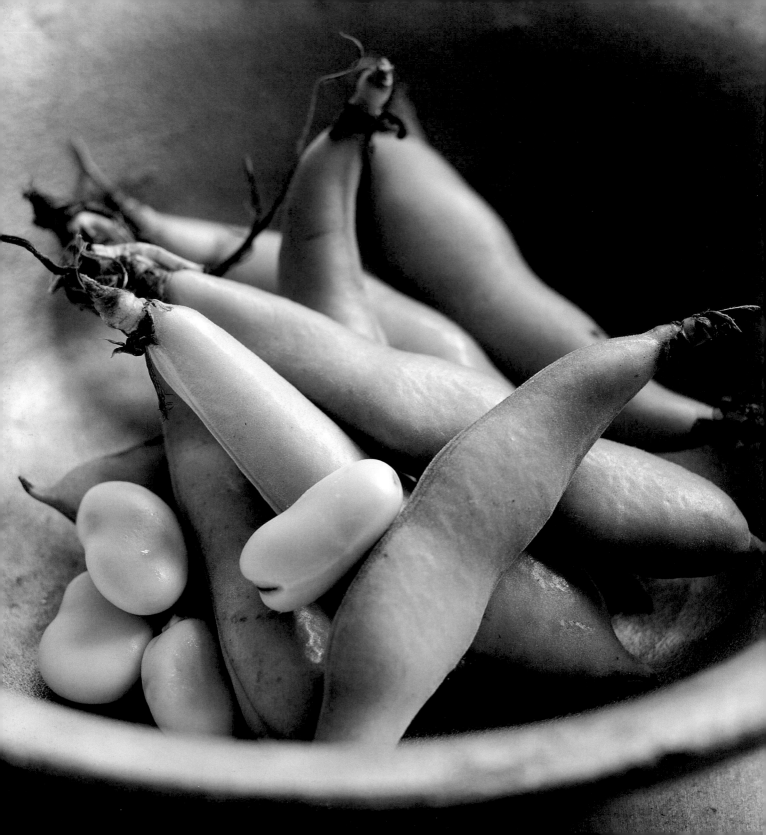

2

soups and salads

Jerusalem artichoke soup

Jerusalem artichokes have nothing to do with Jerusalem or globe artichokes, but are a good part of a healthy diet. They also taste great raw and grated over salads.

Olive-oil spray (see page 17)
450g Jerusalem artichokes, peeled, diced and submerged in acidulated water (water with a little lemon juice or vinegar added)
1 onion, diced
225g floury potatoes, diced
2 garlic cloves, finely chopped
1 celery stick, diced
1 heaped teaspoon soft thyme leaves
1 litre chicken or vegetable stock
150ml skimmed milk
4 tablespoons low-fat Greek yogurt
Pinch of freshly grated nutmeg
50g tender young spinach leaves
Freshly ground black pepper

Serves 4

Lightly spray a pan with olive oil. Drain the artichokes and add them to the pan. Add the onion, potatoes, garlic, celery and thyme, then stir to combine. Cover with a lid and cook for 10 minutes, shaking the pan occasionally, until the potatoes have started to soften but not colour.

Pour the stock into the pan, bring to the boil, then reduce to a simmer and cook for another 10 minutes or so until all the vegetables have softened and are completely tender. Leave to cool a little and then blend in batches using a hand-held mixer or food processor until smooth. If you would like a squeaky-smooth soup, pass through a fine sieve. Return the soup to the pan.

Add the milk and yogurt to the pan, whisk to combine, add the nutmeg and spinach and reheat gently, stirring, until the spinach has wilted. Season with black pepper to taste and ladle into warmed soup bowls. Serve with crusty wholegrain bread.

PER SERVING:
164 KCALS, 2G FAT, 1G SATURATED FAT, 32GCARBOHYDRATE, 0.39G SODIUM

watercress and potato soup

With its abundance of vitamins and minerals, watercress is a real superfood. Combined with potato, this a classic French combination that tastes wonderful. This is warm and thick soup, perfect for the winter months.

2 shallots, finely diced
1 sprig thyme
25g unsalted butter
2 bunches watercress, leaves and stalks separated
325g floury potatoes, diced
1.2 litres vegetable or chicken stock, boiling
4 tablespoons low-fat yogurt
Freshly ground black pepper

Serves 4

In a pan, cook the shallots and thyme gently in the butter until softened but not coloured. Tie the watercress stalks together with string, then put in the pan. Add potatoes and stir to combine.

Add the boiling stock and cook aggressively until the potatoes are soft. Remove the watercress stalks and discard.

Add half the watercress leaves, cook for a further minute, then liquidise in a blender. Pass the puréed soup through a fine sieve. Whisk in the yogurt and the remaining watercress leaves. Heat through and season with black pepper before serving.

PER SERVING:
123 KCALS, 6G FAT, 3G SATURATED FAT, 13G CARBOHYDRATE, 0.43G SODIUM

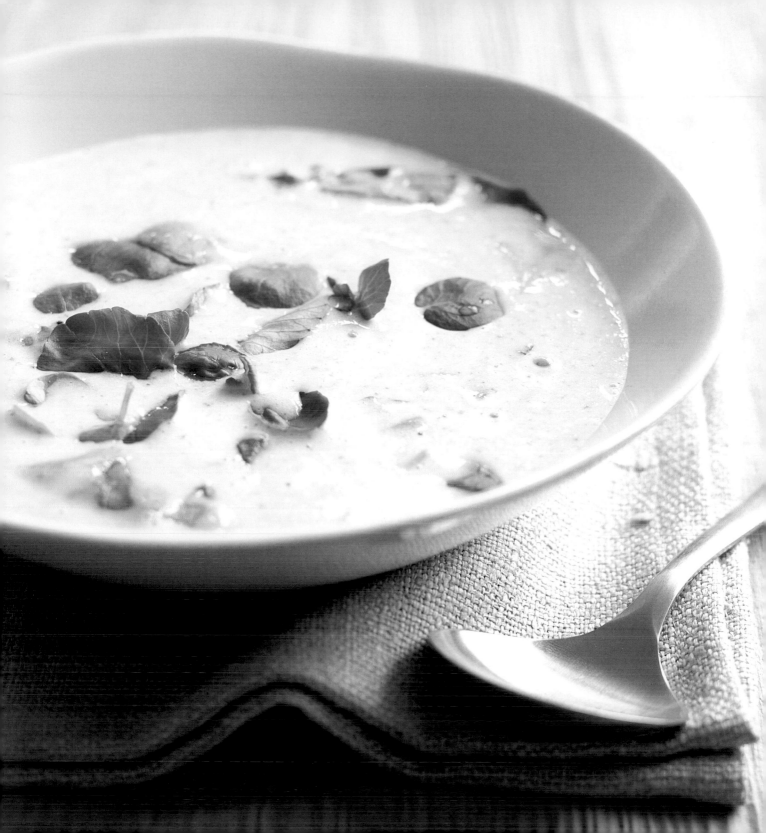

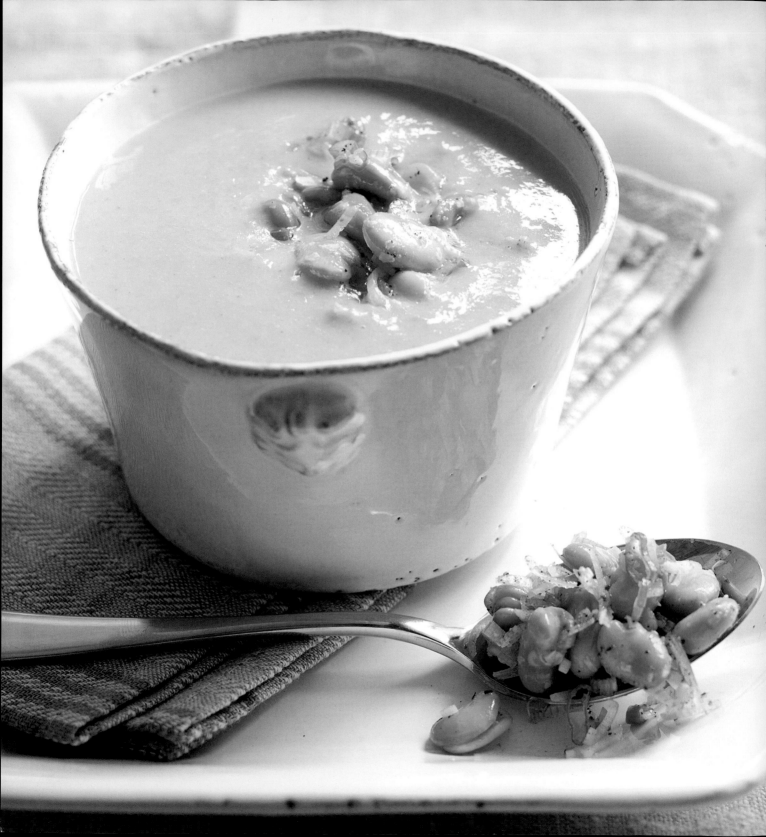

cold pea and mint soup with a broad bean salad

A perfect light summer lunch. Use fresh podded peas when in season, but to be honest, frozen peas are just as tasty and nutritious.

900ml vegetable stock
1 garlic clove, crushed
4 spring onions, sliced
1 tablespoon vegetable oil
450g podded peas
   (fresh or frozen)
1 tablespoon caster sugar
2 tablespoons chopped mint leaves
Freshly ground black pepper
150ml low-fat Greek yogurt

For the broad bean salad
175g broad beans,
   weighed after podding and
   skinning, or 400g tinned
   white beans, drained
4 spring onions, finely sliced
1 tablespoon olive oil
1 teaspoon lemon juice
1 tablespoon grated Parmesan
   cheese

Serves 4

In a saucepan, bring the vegetable stock to the boil.

In a separate saucepan, cook the garlic and spring onions in the vegetable oil until the onion is soft but not brown. Add the peas and sugar, then add the boiling stock. Cook for 12 minutes if you are using fresh peas, 4 minutes if frozen. Allow to cool.

In a liquidiser, blend the soup with the mint. Season with black pepper to taste, cool and refrigerate. When chilled, whisk in the yogurt.

To make the salad, just before serving combine the broad beans or white beans and spring onions with the olive oil and lemon juice. Season with plenty of ground pepper. Fold in the Parmesan.

Make a small pile of the salad in the centre of 4 soup plates, pour the soup around and serve immediately.

PER SERVING:
238 KCALS, 11G FAT, 3G SATURATED FAT, 22G CARBOHYDRATE, 0.35G SODIUM

a warming rustic garlic soup

A soup to lift the heart, garlic is full of beneficial properties. It is antibacterial, and antiviral and may help to reduce blood cholesterol and nasal congestion.

5 garlic cloves, thinly sliced
25g lean streaky bacon, finely diced (optional)
1 red chilli, finely sliced
1 onion, finely sliced
1 teaspoon soft thyme leaves
1 tablespoon olive oil
4 thick slices wholegrain bread, crusts removed
½ teaspoon paprika
600ml chicken stock
Freshly ground black pepper

Serves 2

In a saucepan cook the garlic, bacon, if using, chilli, onion and thyme in the olive oil until golden. Break the bread into small cubes and add to the pan with the paprika and chicken stock.

Bring to the boil and simmer for 10 minutes, stirring from time to time until the bread has broken down and thickened the liquid. For a smoother soup, blend in a liquidiser or food processor. Season with black pepper to taste.

PER SERVING:
271 KCALS, 8G FAT, 1G SATURATED FAT, 42G CARBOHYDRATE, 0.83G SODIUM

toasted pasta in wild mushroom broth

This is the perfect soup to make in autumn or winter when wild mushrooms are at their best. A good source of carbohydrates.

110g wholewheat fettuccine
1 tablespoon olive oil
Olive-oil spray (see page 17)
1 teaspoon soft thyme leaves
1 teaspoon chopped garlic
2 onions, roughly chopped
25g dried ceps or porcini,
    soaked in 300ml boiling water
1 bunch parsley, leaves and stalks

1 teaspoon black peppercorns
1.2 litres vegetable or
    chicken stock
225g mixed fresh wild
    mushrooms, cleaned
50g button mushrooms,
    cleaned
Freshly ground pepper
1 bunch spring onions, sliced

Serves 4

Preheat the oven to 180°/350°F/gas mark 4.

Break the pasta into smaller pieces, toss in the oil and place on a baking sheet. Bake in the oven for 10 minutes until golden. Set aside to cool.

Spray a saucepan with a little olive oil and cook the thyme, garlic and onions over a medium heat for about 10 minutes or until the onion has softened, but not coloured. Add the soaked mushrooms with their liquid, the parsley stalks, peppercorns and the stock, bring to the boil and cook for 30 minutes.

Meanwhile remove any stalks from the wild mushrooms and add them to the stock. Slice the mushroom caps, quarter the button mushrooms and set aside.

Strain the stock, wipe out the saucepan and return the strained liquid to the saucepan. Add the pasta and the prepared fresh mushrooms and cook for a further 10 minutes. Season with black pepper to taste and sprinkle with spring onions. Serve very hot.

PER SERVING:
184 KCALS, 5G FAT, 1G SATURATED FAT, 30G CARBOHYDRATE, 0.47G SODIUM

tomato water

The ultimate slimming soup, this is also highly refreshing and light and well worth the effort. Presentation is everything here: the basil should float elegantly around the small tomato dice. Serve with some wholemeal bread or have as a starter.

1kg ripe but firm vine tomatoes, roughly chopped
1 tablespoon Worcestershire sauce
1 teaspoon Tabasco sauce
½ cucumber, cut into chunks
300ml Evian water
1 teaspoon salt
3 plum tomatoes, seeded and diced
6 basil leaves

Serves 4

Blend all the ingredients, except for the plum tomatoes and basil, in a liquidiser.

Pour the pulp into jelly bags and allow to drip through, preferably overnight. Do not force through as it will cloud the liquid. Chill until ready to serve.

Garnish each bowl with diced tomato and some chiffonade of shredded basil. Pour the tomato water over and serve immediately.

PER SERVING:
64 KCALS, 1G FAT, 0.1G SATURATED FAT, 12G CARBOHYDRATE, 0.59G SODIUM

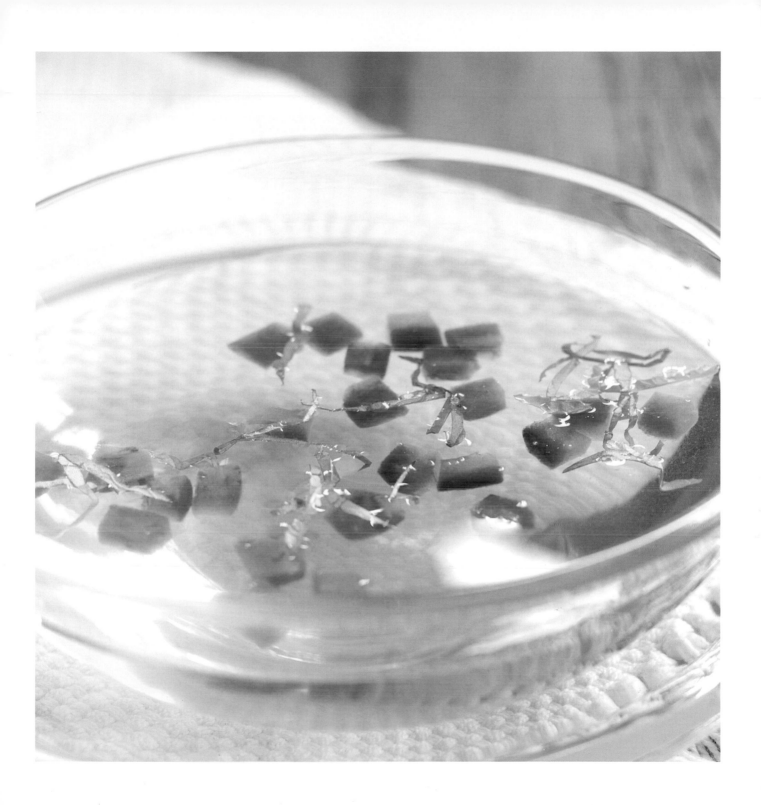

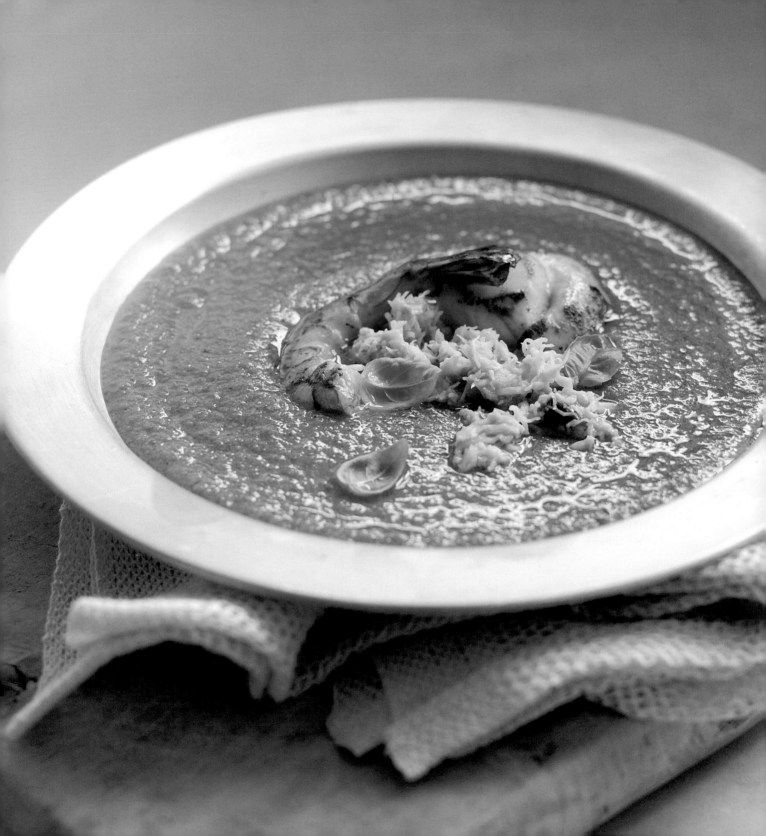

grilled shellfish gazpacho

An exciting variation on a Spanish theme; gazpacho is usually a vegetarian soup, but here I have added prawns, scallops and crab meat. Serve with some wholemeal toast.

1 slice wholegrain country bread, crusts removed and broken into small chunks
1 dessertspoon sherry vinegar
½ garlic clove, finely chopped
1 teaspoon caster sugar
½ red chilli, seeded, finely diced
2 tablespoons olive oil, plus extra for brushing
350g plum tomatoes, peeled and seeded
200ml tomato juice
2 spring onions, finely sliced

½ red pepper, roasted or grilled, peeled, seeded and diced
½ large cucumber, peeled, seeded and roughly diced
1 dessertspoon pesto
Freshly ground black pepper
3 large raw prawns, shelled
4 diver-caught scallops, shucked
Basil leaves to garnish
125g white crab meat
For the basil salt (optional)
Handful of basil leaves
125g Maldon salt

Serves 4

Place the bread in a food processor or blender. While blitzing, add the vinegar, garlic, sugar and chilli and blend until smooth.

Add the olive oil, a little at a time, until it has been absorbed by the bread. Add the tomatoes, tomato juice, spring onions, red pepper, cucumber and pesto. Continue to blitz until a smooth emulsion is formed. Season to taste with black pepper.

To make the basil salt, place the ingredients in a food processor and blend until smooth and green. Store in an airtight container. Half an hour before serving, sprinkle prawns and scallops with ½ teaspoon of the basil salt, if desired, and toss to combine.

Dust off the salt from the prawns and scallops and brush with a little olive oil. Cook them under a hot grill or in a griddle or heavy-based frying pan for 1–2 minutes on each side. Ideally serve in large-rimmed shallow soup bowls. Place the prawns and scallops in the centre, then pour the soup around the shellfish. Scatter each bowl with basil leaves and fresh crab and serve immediately.

PER SERVING:
198 KCALS, 10G FAT, 2G SATURATED FAT, 11G CARBOHYDRATE, 0.65G SODIUM

poached shellfish in oriental broth

Another seafood speciality, this soup contains light, vibrant flavours, but with a little bite. A recipe with lots of Asian tastes. Serve with wholemeal bread.

1 tablespoon vegetable oil
1 teaspoon Thai red curry paste
2 garlic cloves, sliced
1 onion, thinly sliced
½ fennel head, thinly sliced
1 tablespoon tomato purée
1 lemongrass stalk, finely chopped
2 dried bird's eye chillies
1 kaffir lime leaf, shredded (optional)
1cm piece of fresh root ginger, finely chopped
1 'petal' broken off a star anise
2 litres fish stock
1 teaspoon chopped tarragon

For finishing the broth
110g asparagus tips
50g podded peas (fresh or frozen)
4 large diver-caught scallops
110g salmon fillet, cut into 4 pieces
8 large shelled prawns, peeled and deveined
24 mussels, cleaned
110g white crab meat
75g sugar-snap peas
2 tomatoes, quartered and seeded
Juice of 2 limes
1 tablespoon nam pla (Thai fish sauce)
24 coriander leaves
Handful of baby spinach leaves

Serves 4

Heat the oil in a saucepan, add the curry paste and cook for 1 minute, stirring regularly. Add the garlic, onion and fennel and cook gently for 10 minutes.

Stir in the tomato purée, lemongrass, chillies, lime leaf (if using), ginger and star anise. Pour on the stock and add the tarragon. Simmer over a low heat for an hour, then strain the broth into a clean saucepan.

Bring the broth to the boil, add the asparagus and peas and cook for 2 minutes. Add the scallops and salmon and cook for a further 2 minutes. Add the remaining ingredients and cook until the mussels have opened. Ladle into 4 warm bowls.

PER SERVING.
241 KCALS, 9G FAT, 1G SATURATED FAT, 10G CARBOHYDRATE, 1.26G SODIUM

a thai soup of whiting and squid

Whiting is an underused fish that is suited to Thai flavours. If you can't find it, you can use cod, haddock or monkfish instead.

1.5 litres fish stock
1 lime, thinly sliced
2 kaffir lime leaves, finely shredded
3 garlic cloves, crushed
3 red chillies, thinly sliced
2½cm piece of fresh root ginger, sliced
1 lemongrass stalk, finely chopped
2 tablespoons nam pla (Thai fish sauce)
450g whiting fillets, cut into 5cm cubes
225g baby asparagus tips
4 spring onions, sliced
450g squid tubes, cut into 5cm cubes
175g sugar-snap peas
Freshly ground black pepper
2 tablespoons chopped coriander leaves

Serves 6

In a large saucepan, bring the stock to the boil and add the lime, lime leaves, garlic, chillies, ginger, lemongrass and nam pla. Simmer for 5 minutes.

Add the whiting, asparagus and spring onions and cook for a further 4 minutes. Then add the squid and peas and cook for just 1 more minute. Season with black pepper, garnish with the coriander leaves and serve immediately.

PER SERVING:
159 KCALS, 2G FAT, 0.1G SATURATED FAT, 5G CARBOHYDRATE, 0.83G SODIUM

chicken noodle soup

This version of a classic Chinese soup uses buckwheat noodles instead of egg noodles. As the soup contains plenty of carbs, it is best eaten as a main meal.

225g buckwheat noodles
1 teaspoon sesame oil
1 teaspoon vegetable oil
½ teaspoon grated fresh root ginger
1 garlic clove, finely chopped
½ teaspoon chilli, diced
3 spring onions, sliced
4 tablespoons reduced-salt soy sauce
2 teaspoon runny honey
1.2 litres chicken stock
Freshly ground black pepper
175g cooked chicken, shredded
1 tablespoon chopped coriander leaves

Serves 4

Cook the noodles in boiling water until tender: this should take about 4 minutes. When the noodles are cooked, drain and refresh in cold water.

Meanwhile, in a saucepan, heat both the oils over a medium heat. Add the ginger, garlic, chilli and spring onions and cook for 3 minutes, stirring constantly. Add the soy sauce, honey and chicken stock, then bring to the boil and simmer for 3 minutes. Season with black pepper to taste.

Add the noodles to the soup, then add the cooked chicken and coriander. Reheat for 2 minutes before serving.

PER SERVING:
326 KCALS, 7G FAT, 1G SATURATED FAT, 47G CARBOHYDRATE, 1.06G SODIUM

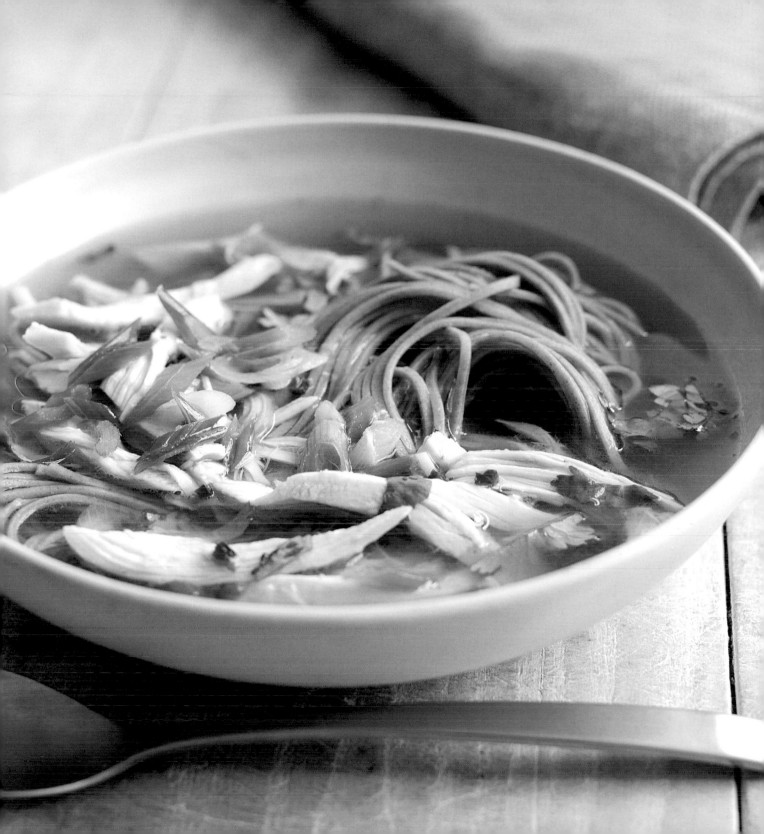

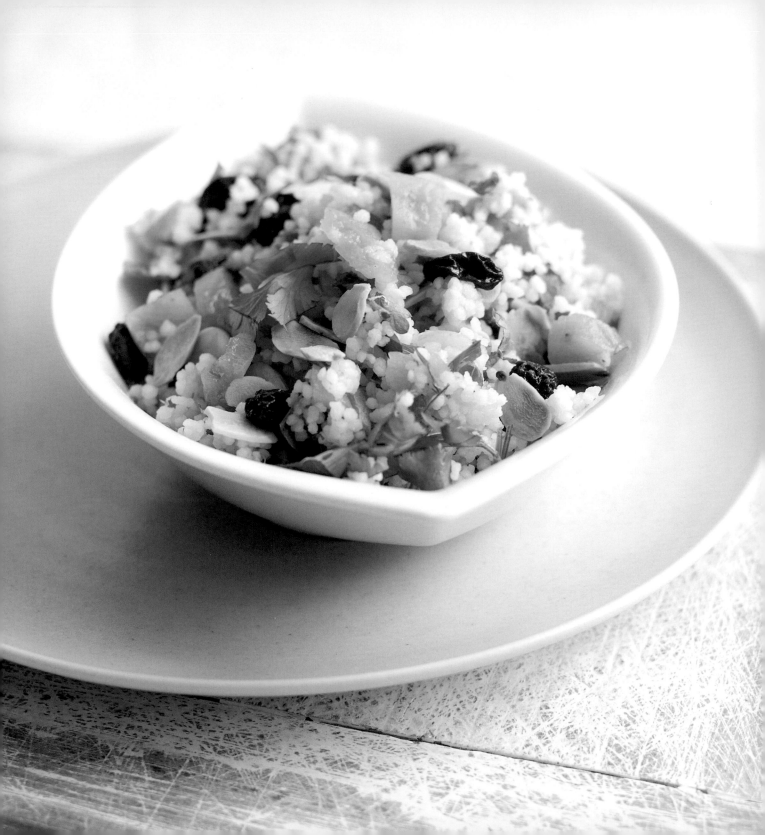

jewelled couscous

Usually an accompaniment to a Moroccan tagine, but it makes a delicious salad too. A version can also be made with rice. Either way, it is a light and colourful dish, rich in flavours.

200ml chicken or vegetable stock
1 tablespoon olive oil
½ teaspoon salt
110g couscous
Finely grated zest of 1 unwaxed lemon
Juice of ½ lemon
25g flaked almonds, toasted
50g dried apricots, soaked in a little water for 20 minutes, drained and chopped
25g sultanas or raisins
4 tablespoons roughly chopped flat-leaf parsley
4 tablespoons roughly chopped coriander

Serves 2

Heat the stock in a large pan with the olive oil and the salt. Bring to the boil and immediately remove from the heat. Pour in the couscous in a thin, steady stream and then stir in the lemon zest. Set aside for 10 minutes to allow the grains to swell and until the couscous has soaked up all of the liquid.

Return the couscous to the heat and drizzle over the lemon juice. Heat gently for about 5 minutes, stirring with a long-pronged fork to fluff up the grains, then remove from the heat.

Fold in the almonds, apricots, sultanas or raisins, parsley and coriander. Season with black pepper to taste. Serve with Chicken Tagine (see page 115) or allow to cool to room temperature and serve as a healthy salad.

PER SERVING:
343 KCALS, 14G FAT, 1G SATURATED FAT, 49G CARBOHYDRATE, 0.64G SODIUM

butternut squash salad with garlic, chilli and caraway

Butternut squash are a good source of beta-carotene and vitamin E. They can be used in sweet or savoury dishes and are often cooked with spices.

1 medium-sized butternut squash, cut into wedges
6 garlic cloves
Freshly ground black pepper
1 teaspoon thyme leaves
2 tablespoons olive oil
1 tablespoon balsamic vinegar
1 tablespoon red wine vinegar
1 tablespoon harissa
1½ teaspoons ground caraway seeds
2 tablespoons chopped coriander leaves
2 eggs, hard-boiled, peeled and quartered

Serves 4

Preheat the oven to 180°C/350°F/gas mark 4.

Place the squash in a roasting dish, cut side up, and add the garlic cloves. Sprinkle with pepper and half the olive oil. Roast for about 40 minutes or until soft and golden, turning from time to time. Remove from the oven and allow to cool to room temperature.

Scrape the butternut pulp from the skin and mash together with the garlic and any juices from the roasting dish. Fold in the remaining ingredients except for the eggs.

Place in a bowl and garnish with the eggs before serving.

PER SERVING:
157 KCALS, 10G FAT, 2G SATURATED FAT, 12G CARBOHYDRATE, 0.06G SODIUM

salsa verde

A light, refreshing side dish, this also makes a great accompaniment to meat dishes such as the Bacon Bollito on page 120. The pickled cucumber, lemon juice and vinegar give this a surprising kick.

1 handful flat-leaf parsley leaves
6 basil leaves
1 pickled cucumber, roughly chopped
1½ garlic cloves, roughly chopped
1 tablespoon capers, drained and rinsed
2 tinned anchovy fillets, drained and rinsed
½ tablespoon red wine vinegar
½ tablespoon lemon juice
3 tablespoons extra virgin olive oil
½ tablespoon Dijon mustard
Pinch of freshly ground black pepper

Serves 4

Coarsely chop together the herbs, cucumber, garlic, capers and anchovies or pulse in a food processor. (You get a better result if you hand-chop this salsa.)

Transfer the mixture to a non-reactive bowl and slowly add the remaining ingredients whilst whisking.

PER SERVING:
87 KCALS, 9G FAT, 1G SATURATED FAT, 1G CARBOHYDRATE, 0.29G SODIUM

button mushroom and baby spinach salad

A salad with attitude, and one for the waistline. This light dish is perfect for summer picnics or as an accompaniment to a main course.

110g button mushrooms, cleaned and quartered
Pinch of salt
3 tablespoons lemon juice
½ teaspoon powdered rosemary
2 tablespoons roughly chopped flat-leaf parsley
2 teaspoons olive oil
3 tablespoons low-fat Greek yogurt
2 tablespoons skimmed milk
Freshly ground black pepper
2 handfuls baby spinach
2 tablespoons snipped chives

Serves 2

Place the mushrooms in a large bowl, sprinkle with a little salt and leave for 30 minutes. Rinse under cold water and dry with kitchen paper.

Combine the lemon juice, rosemary, parsley and olive oil and spoon over the mushrooms, then toss to combine.

Thin the yogurt with a little milk and pour over the mushrooms. Season with black pepper to taste.

Divide the spinach between 2 plates, spoon the mushrooms into the centre of the spinach and sprinkle with the chives.

PER SERVING:
75 KCALS, 5G FAT, 1G SATURATED FAT, 4G CARBOHYDRATE, 0.48G SODIUM

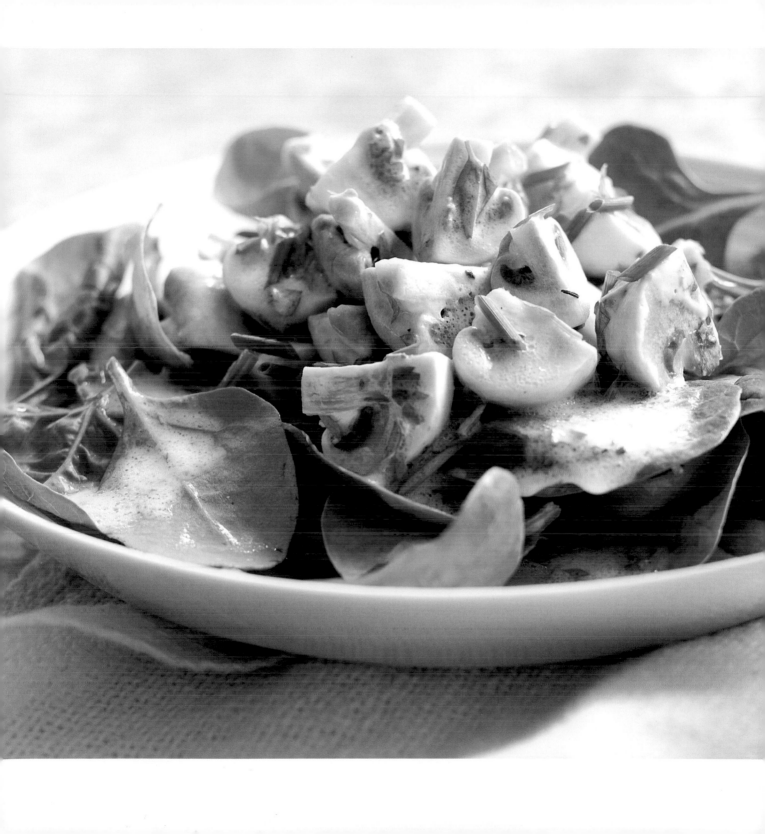

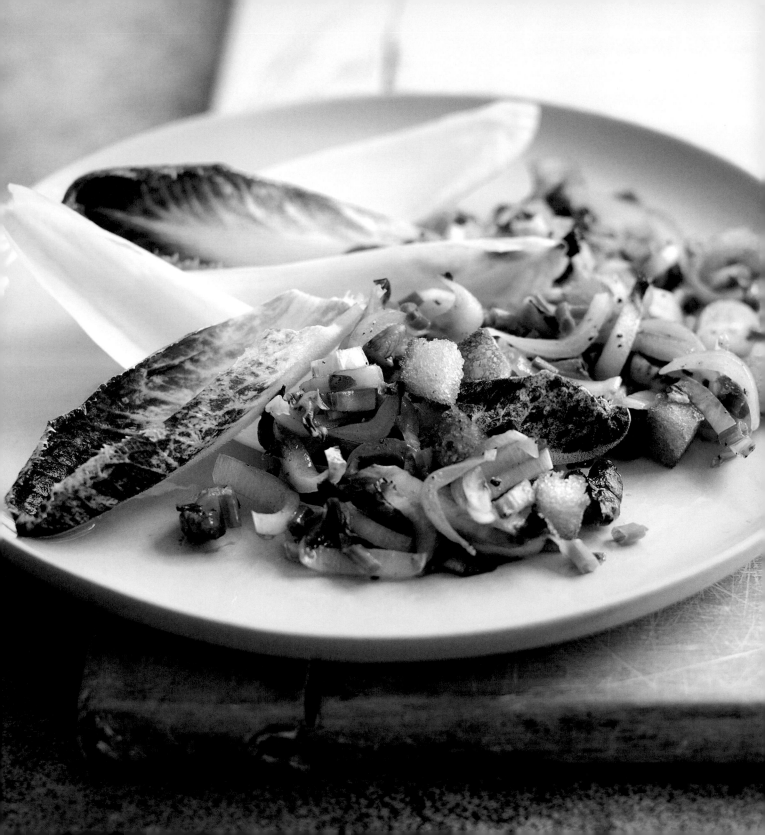

chicory salad with walnuts and croûtons

The slightly bitter taste of the chicory is offset by the nuts and sweet vinegar. Although this is relatively high in fat, most of it is unsaturated.

2 heads chicory or Belgian endive
Olive-oil spray (see page 17)
1 garlic clove, diced
1 slice country bread, cut into croûtons
½ tablespoon walnut oil
4 walnuts, roughly chopped
1 tablespoon aged sherry vinegar
Freshly ground black pepper
2 tablespoons chopped chives

Serves 2

Separate the leaves from the chicory, and wash if necessary. Retaining a dozen larger whole leaves, shred the remainder, then set aside.

Lightly spray a frying pan with olive oil. Heat, then add the garlic and the croûtons and fry until golden. Add the shredded chicory, walnut oil and walnuts. Cook for 1 minute and then add the sherry vinegar. Season with black pepper to taste.

Arrange 6 whole chicory leaves around each plate and place the warm chicory salad in the centre. Serve immediately.

PER SERVING:
203 KCALS, 13G FAT, 1G SATURATED FAT, 17G CARBOHYDRATE, 0.14G SODIUM

seared scallops on avocado, beetroot and orange salad

Lovely colours, lovely textures and a little luxury. Choose diver-caught scallops rather than dredged as dredging damages the sea bed.

Juice and grated zest of 1 orange
Juice and grated zest of 1 lime
1 tablespoon walnut oil
½ tablespoon olive oil
1 shallot, finely diced
Freshly ground black pepper
2 small cooked, but not pickled, beetroot, cut into 1cm dice
2 naval oranges, peeled, pith removed and sliced horizontally into 5
½ avocado, peeled and diced
4 large diver-caught scallops
Olive-oil spray (see page 17)
2 teaspoons chopped dill

Serves 2

Whisk together the juice and zest of the orange and lime, walnut oil, the olive oil and shallot and season with black pepper to taste. Add the beetroot and leave for a couple of hours until the dressing has taken on a beautiful shade of red.

Arrange half the orange slices on each plate and scatter over the diced avocado.

Season the scallops with black pepper. Heat a non-stick frying pan over a high flame and lightly spray with olive oil. Add the scallops and cook for 1½ minutes on each side until crusty and golden, but still a little opaque in the centre. Just before serving, spoon the beetroot with its dressing over the avocado, top each plate with 2 scallops and garnish with dill.

PER SERVING:
270 KCALS, 16G FAT, 2G SATURATED FAT, 19G CARBOHYDRATE, 0.15G SODIUM

spicy sardines with chickpea and avocado salad

A great Mediterranean combo that is just as good made with tinned sardines. Sardines and chickpeas are also full of goodness. Serve as a main meal.

Olive-oil spray (see page 17)
1 red chilli, diced
2 shallots, diced
1 tablespoon finely chopped flat-leaf parsley
1 tablespoon finely chopped coriander leaves
3 garlic cloves, crushed
8 sardines, scaled, cleaned, flattened out and head and backbone removed
Juice of 1 lemon

Serves 4

For the chickpea and avocado salad
Yolk of 1 hard-boiled egg
3 tablespoons olive oil
2 tablespoons red wine vinegar
½ red onion, finely chopped
1 garlic clove, crushed
2 tablespoons chopped parsley
1 tablespoon small capers, drained and rinsed
400g tinned chickpeas, drained and rinsed
1 ripe avocado, peeled and chopped into chunky dice
Pinch of salt
Freshly ground black pepper

To make the salad, place the egg yolk in a bowl, beat in the oil and vinegar and stir in the onion, garlic, parsley, capers, chickpeas and avocado. Season with salt and black pepper.

Preheat the oven to 180°C/350°F/gas mark 4.

Lightly spray a small frying pan with olive-oil spray, then add the chilli and shallots and cook until softened but not coloured. Fold in the parsley, coriander and garlic and season with black pepper, then spread over the flesh side of the fish.

Roll up the sardines and secure with 2 small wooden cocktail sticks that have been soaked in water. Cook in the oven for 5–8 minutes, then place the sardines on a plate and drizzle with lemon juice.

To serve, place a pile of salad on to each serving plate and top with two sardine rolls.

PER SERVING:
407 KCALS, 28G FAT, 4G SATURATED FAT, 13G CARBOHYDRATE, 0.45G SODIUM

mediterranean seafood salad

A special balance of flavours in a healthy package. The Mediterranean diet is one of the healthiest in the world, with its combination of fresh fish, olive oil and colourful vegetables.

125ml dry white wine
1kg mussels, cleaned
6 squid tubes, cut into rings
18 raw tiger prawns, peeled
6 diver-caught scallops, halved
175g tinned cockles or baby clams, shelled and drained
125g cooked white crab meat

3 garlic cloves, crushed
2 red chillies, finely sliced
½ red onion, diced
3 tablespoons olive oil
1 tablespoon lemon juice
Freshly ground black pepper
2 tablespoons chopped flat-leaf parsley
Crisp lettuce

Serves 6

In a large saucepan, bring the white wine to the boil, add the mussels, cover and cook for 5 minutes or until the mussels have opened. Remove the mussels from the pan and set aside, reserving the liquid. Discard any that remain closed. Shell the mussels when cool enough to handle.

In the boiling juices that remain in the pan, cook the squid, prawns and scallops for 1 minute. Remove (do not throw away the cooking liquid), allow the shellfish to cool and combine with the mussels, cockles or clams and white crab meat.

Boil the mussel cooking liquid until it has reduced to about 4 tablespoons. Combine with the garlic, chillies, onion, olive oil and lemon juice. Pour the juices over the seafood and toss to combine. Refrigerate for 30 minutes, season with black pepper and fold in the chopped parsley.

Serve on a bed of crisp lettuce with some warm crusty wholegrain bread to mop up the juices.

PER SERVING:
243 KCALS, 9G FAT, 1G SATURATED FAT, 4G CARBOHYDRATE, 0.46G SODIUM

warm salad of asparagus, field mushrooms and peas

Something a little different, this is a wonderful spring dish, when asparagus and fresh peas are in season.

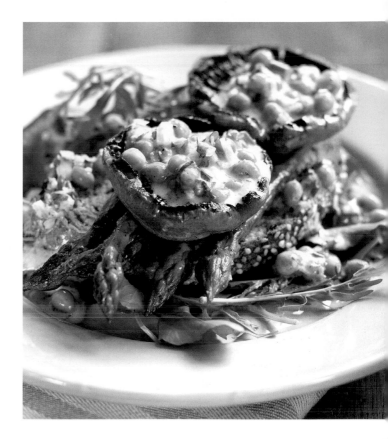

10 medium asparagus spears, trimmed and peeled if necessary
75g podded young peas
2 tablespoons olive oil
1 garlic clove, mashed to a paste
4 field mushrooms, stalks removed, peeled if necessary
Freshly ground black pepper
2 slices wholemeal bread
½ shallot, finely chopped
3 tablespoons dry Martini (optional)
2 tablespoons low-fat yogurt
½ tablespoon chopped flat leaf parsley
½ tablespoon snipped chives
½ teaspoon chopped tarragon
½ tablespoon lemon juice
½ handful rocket
½ handful watercress

Serves 2

Cook the asparagus in boiling water for 1 minute, drain, reserving the cooking water, and set aside.

Add the peas to the asparagus cooking water and cook for 2 minutes, drain, then set aside.

Prepare your barbecue, grill or griddle pan.

Combine the olive oil and garlic and brush over the asparagus and the mushrooms. Season the asparagus and mushrooms with black pepper.

Grill or barbecue the mushrooms for 5 minutes on each side and the asparagus for 2 minutes each side. Keep both warm. Brush both sides of the bread with garlic-infused oil and grill until both sides are toasted.

In a saucepan, heat the remaining garlic oil, add the shallot, and over a medium heat allow to cook without colouring. Add the dry Martini, if using, increase the heat and cook for a further minute. Remove the pan from the heat and whisk in the yogurt a little at a time. Fold in the peas, parsley, chives, tarragon and lemon juice. Season to taste. Return to a gentle heat to warm through.

Combine the rocket and watercress and divide between 2 plates. Top the leaves with a slice of the grilled bread. Divide the asparagus and mushrooms between the bread slices, arranging them attractively on top of each slice. Spoon the peas and juices over the salad leaves.

PER SERVING:
261 KCALS, 14G FAT, 2G SATURATED FAT, 24G CARBOHYDRATE, 0.22G SODIUM

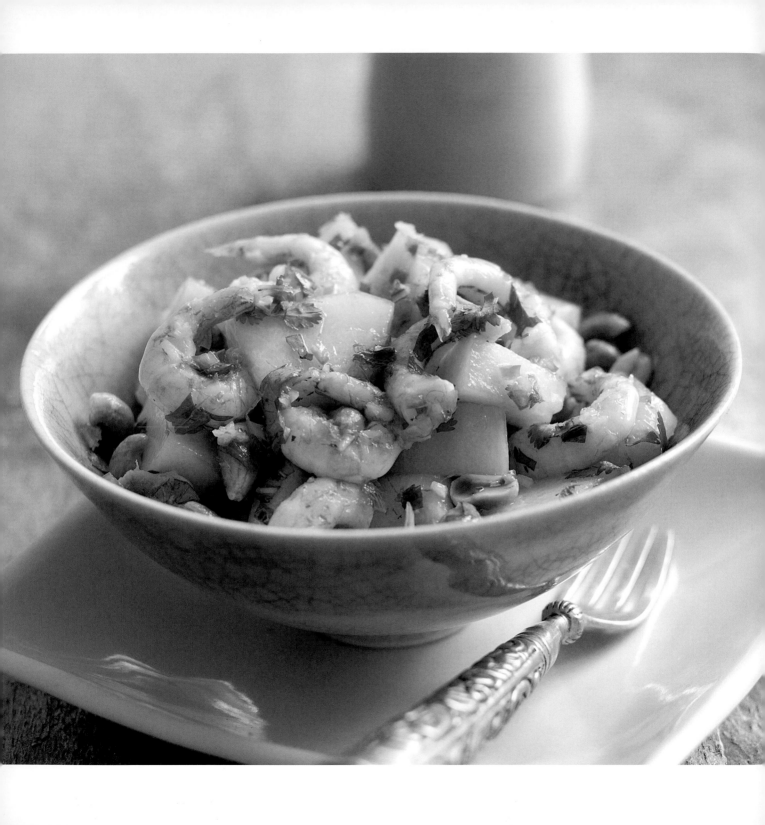

thai-inspired melon salad

This salad was created as a result of my visits to Thailand. Their vibrant flavours go well with melon, creating a refreshing salad with a twist. As this is a salty salad, keep the rest of the day's intake low.

2 garlic cloves, crushed
1 tablespoon runny honey
2 teaspoons nam pla (Thai fish sauce)
Juice of 2 limes
1 tablespoon grated lime zest
2 red chillies, finely diced
175g cooked and shelled shrimp or prawns
50g unsalted roasted peanuts
1 Galia or Ogen melon, peeled and chopped into 2.5cm dice
4 tablespoons chopped coriander leaves
1 tablespoon chopped mint leaves

Serves 4

In a large bowl, combine the garlic, honey, nam pla, lime juice, lime zest and chillies. Fold in the shrimp and peanuts. Add the melon and stir to combine.

Garnish with chopped coriander and mint. Chill until ready to serve.

PER SERVING:
162 KCALS, 7G FAT, 1G SATURATED FAT, 10G CARBOHYDRATE, 1.87G SODIUM

prawn and sweetcorn salad

This is the salad for those in a hurry. Just chuck it all together in a bowl to create a healthy meal in minutes. Quick, simple and exceedingly tasty.

1 egg yolk
2 tablespoons olive oil
1 tablespoon lemon juice
½ tablespoon Dijon mustard
2 tablespoons low-fat Greek yogurt
2 tablespoons snipped chives
2 tablespoons snipped dill
1 tablespoon sliced spring onion
12 frozen prawns, cooked
175g fresh or frozen sweetcorn kernels, cooked

Serves 2

Whisk together the egg yolk, oil, lemon juice and mustard. Once this has emulsified, fold in the yogurt.

Add the herbs and spring onion and combine with the prawns and sweetcorn.

PER SERVING:
426 KCALS, 19G FAT, 3G SATURATED FAT, 18G CARBOHYDRATE, 1.57G SODIUM

rare tuna salade niçoise

This was inspired by the classic salade niçoise, which uses tinned tuna. Fresh tuna, of course, contains lots of beneficial omega-3 fatty oils. Eat as a main course with crusty bread.

2 x 100g fresh tuna steaks, each ideally 2.5cm thick
4 new salad potatoes
2 eggs, at room temperature
50g extra-fine French beans, trimmed
2 Little Gem lettuce hearts, quartered lengthways and separated into leaves
2 plum tomatoes, roughly chopped
½ red onion, finely sliced
4 tinned anchovy fillets, drained, rinsed and cut lengthways into thin strips
10 black olives, pitted
8 basil leaves, torn

For the marinade
2 tablespoons olive oil
1 tablespoon aged red wine vinegar
1 tablespoon chopped flat-leaf parsley
1 tablespoon snipped chives
1 garlic clove, finely chopped
Freshly ground black pepper

Serves 2

To make the marinade, place the olive oil, vinegar, parsley, chives, garlic and a teaspoon of pepper in a bowl, and whisk to combine.

Place the tuna in a shallow non-metallic dish and pour over half of the marinade. Cover with clingfilm and chill for 1 hour to allow the flavours to penetrate the tuna, turning after about 30 minutes or so.

Place the potatoes in a pan of boiling water, cover and simmer for 10–12 minutes or until just tender. Drain, then cut into quarters lengthways.

Place the eggs in a small pan and just cover with boiling water, then cook for 6 minutes. Drain and rinse under cold running water, remove the shells and cut each egg in half; they should still be slightly soft. Plunge the French beans in a pan of boiling water and blanch for 3 minutes or so, then drain and refresh in cold water.

Heat a griddle pan for 5 minutes. Remove the tuna from the marinade, shaking off any excess. Cook the tuna for about 2 minutes on each side, depending on how rare you like it.

Arrange the lettuce leaves on serving plates or on 1 large platter and add the potatoes, French beans, tomatoes, onion and anchovies. Place the tuna steaks on top and drizzle over the remaining marinade. Scatter over the eggs, olives and torn basil leaves to serve.

PER SERVING:
442 KCALS, 25G FAT, 5G SATURATED FAT, 21G CARBOHYDRATE, 0.71G SODIUM

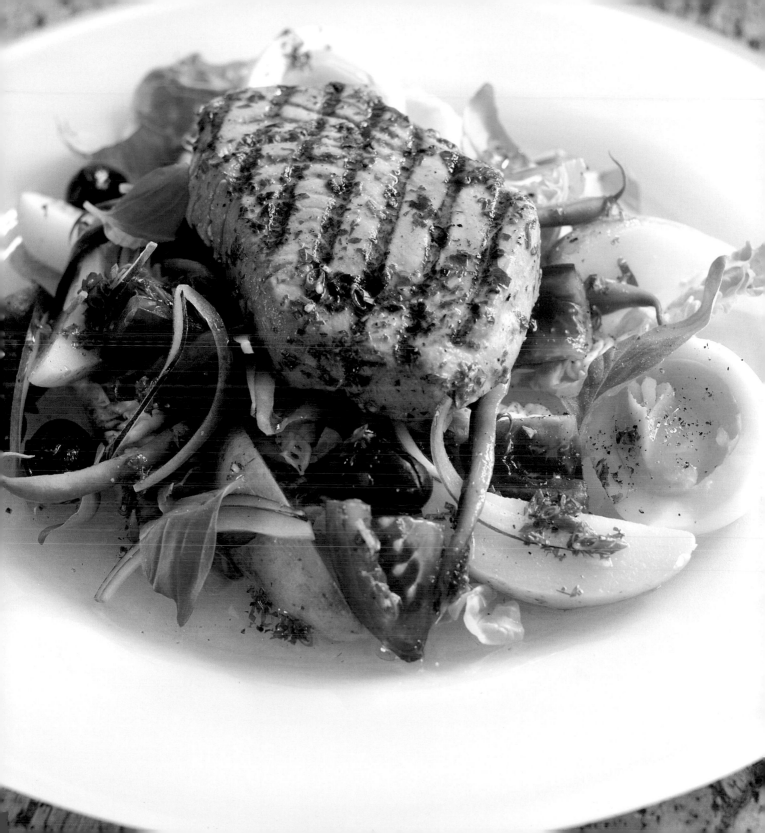

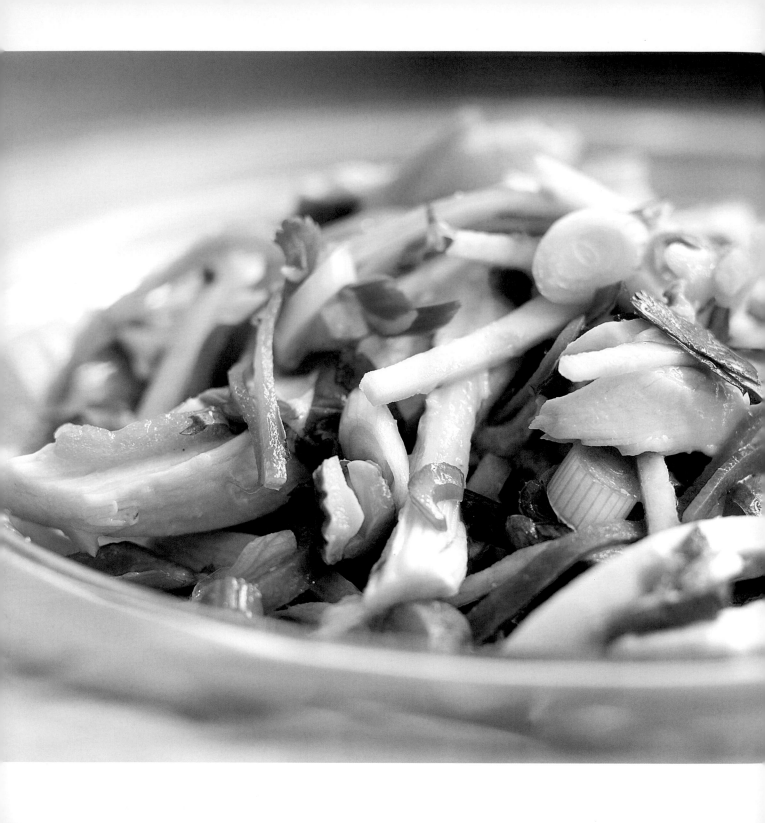

asian chicken salad

With the great flavours of the Orient – papaya, coriander, mint, chilli and lime – this is a simple salad to make, but full of flavour. Perfect for a light lunch or as an appetiser. Serve with pitta bread.

450g shredded chicken from 'The Really Useful Chicken' recipe (see page 116)
1 carrot, cut into julienne
½ green paw-paw or papaya, peeled and cut into julienne
3 tablespoons chopped mint
3 tablespoons chopped coriander leaves
1 bunch spring onions, sliced
½ celeriac, cut into julienne
25g unsalted peanuts, roughly chopped
Freshly ground black pepper

For the dressing
2 teaspoons finely chopped garlic
1 tablespoon finely chopped chilli
150ml lime juice
2 tablespoons nam pla (Thai fish sauce) or reduced-salt light soy sauce
1 tablespoon runny honey

Serves 4

To make the dressing, combine the ingredients in a bowl.

In another large bowl, mix the remaining ingredients with enough of the dressing to coat and season well with black pepper to taste.

PER SERVING:
297 KCALS, 12G FAT, 3G SATURATED FAT, 12G CARBOHYDRATE, 0.69G SODIUM

asian slaw

A healthier alternative to normal mayonnaise-based coleslaw, this recipe again draws on the delicious tastes of the Far East, where the diet is low in saturated fat that the Western world would do well to follow. Serve with pitta bread.

225g pak choi, shredded
125g carrots, cut into julienne
4 shallots, sliced
½ tablespoon grated fresh root ginger
2 tablespoons shredded basil leaves
2 tablespoons coriander leaves
1 tablespoon mint leaves
1 garlic clove, chopped
1 hot chilli, seeded and finely chopped
Juice and grated zest of 1 orange
Juice of 2 limes
1 tablespoon nam pla (Thai fish sauce)
½ teaspoon sugar
2 tablespoons groundnut oil
Freshly ground black pepper
1 tablespoon crushed roasted peanuts

Serves 2

Mix the pak choi in a bowl with the carrots, shallots, ginger, basil, coriander, mint, garlic, chilli and orange zest.

In a small bowl, whisk together the orange juice, lime juice, nam pla and sugar. Slowly whisk in the oil until emulsified. Add the dressing to the pak choi and toss well. Season with pepper. Cover and chill for 2–6 hours.

Serve with pitta breads and a sprinkling of crushed roasted peanuts.

PER SERVING:
222 KCALS, 16G FAT, 3G SATURATED FAT, 16G CARBOHYDRATE, 0.82G SODIUM

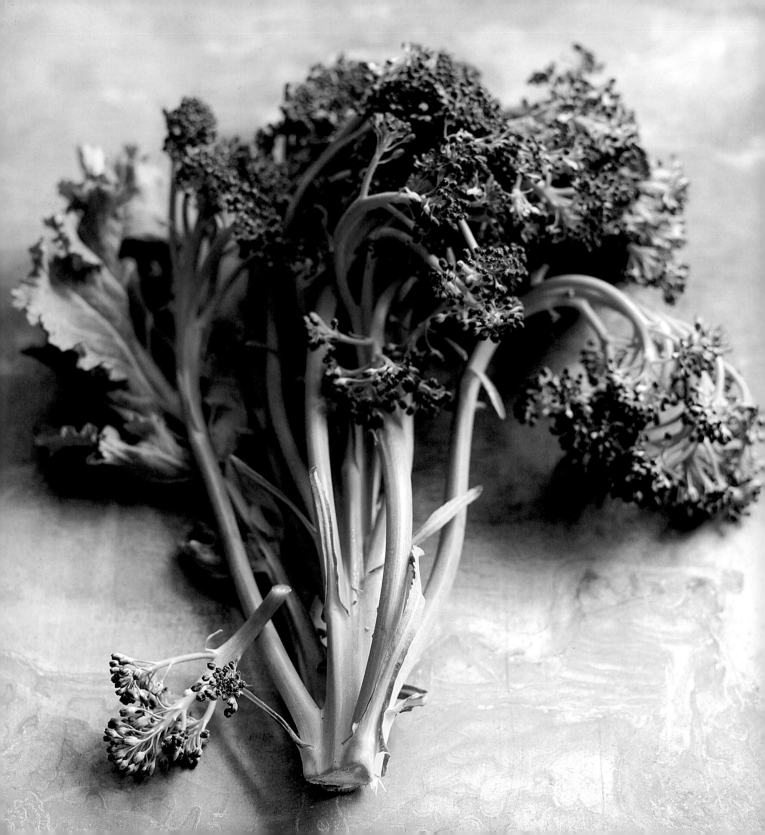

3

light meals
and appetisers

mushroom 'caviar'

An excellent alternative to the usual range of dips, and much healthier. Although the texture may resemble caviar, it has nothing to do with fish or fish roe!

1 tablespoon olive oil
½ onion, finely diced
2 garlic cloves, finely diced
1 teaspoon thyme leaves
100g field mushrooms, roughly chopped
1 tablespoon balsamic vinegar
Freshly ground black pepper

Serves 4

Heat the oil in a deep saucepan over a medium heat. Add the onion, garlic and thyme and cook until soft but not brown.

Add the mushrooms, stir to combine, and increase the heat. Cook for 10 minutes, or until the mushrooms have released their liquid. Then add the balsamic vinegar and cook until all the liquid has evaporated. Season with black pepper to taste.

Blend the mixture in a food processor until roughly chopped but not pulverised. Serve warm or at room temperature with crusty wholegrain bread or oatcakes.

PER SERVING:
39 KCALS, 3G FAT, 0.4G SATURATED FAT, 3G CARBOHYDRATE, 0G SODIUM

asparagus with red pepper sauce

The red peppers add a natural sweetness to the asparagus, a great partnership and fantastic combination of colours. Eat as an appetiser or to accompany a main course.

2 red peppers, seeded and roughly chopped
1 onion, roughly chopped
2 garlic cloves, crushed
1 red chilli, finely diced
12 basil leaves, plus extra to garnish
1 tablespoon walnut oil
1 tablespoon sherry vinegar
2 tablespoons lemon juice
300g asparagus, trimmed
Freshly ground black pepper

Serves 4

Place all the ingredients except the asparagus in a large, non-reactive (not aluminium) saucepan, cover and simmer gently for 20 minutes, stirring from time to time.

Pour the softened pepper mix into a food processor and blend until smooth. Pass through a fine sieve and set aside, keeping it warm, if you wish.

Cook the asparagus in boiling water for 6 minutes, then drain.

Spoon the red pepper sauce (hot or cold) on to 4 plates and top with the asparagus. Garnish with basil leaves and ground black pepper.

PER SERVING:
79 KCALS, 4G FAT, 0.3G SATURATED FAT, 9G CARBOHYDRATE, 0.01G SODIUM

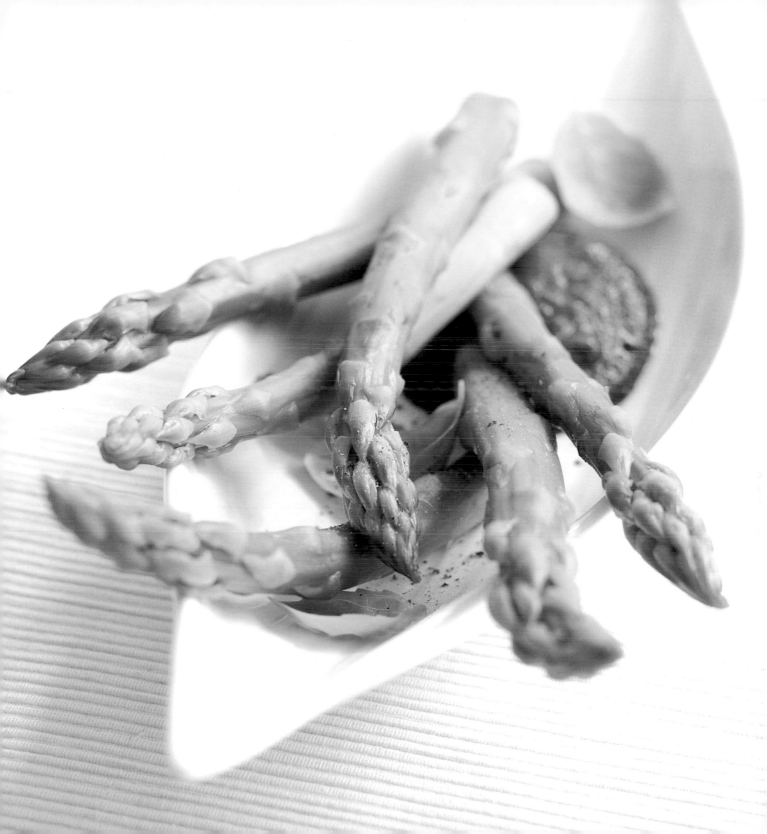

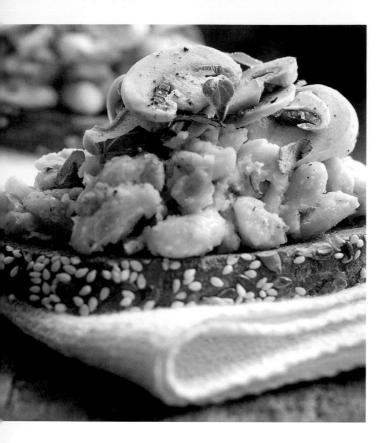

bruschetta with white bean purée and raw mushrooms

A much healthier version of a classic dish, this has lots of fibre and even more flavour.

2 tablespoons olive oil
2 garlic cloves, 1 of them finely diced, 1 halved
1 teaspoon finely chopped rosemary leaves
425g tinned cannellini beans, rinsed and drained
150ml vegetable stock
Freshly ground black pepper
50g button mushrooms, cleaned and sliced
Juice of ½ lemon
1 tablespoon chopped oregano leaves
4 thick slices wholegrain country bread

Serves 4

In a saucepan, combine 1 tablespoon of the olive oil, the diced garlic and the rosemary and cook over a gentle heat until the garlic is soft but without colour.

Add the beans and stock, stir to combine, then cook for about 10 minutes. If the mixture dries out too much, add a little more vegetable stock to moisten. Mash with a potato masher or pulse in a food processor to create a rough purée. Season to taste with ground black pepper.

Meanwhile toss the sliced mushrooms with the remaining olive oil, the lemon juice, oregano and some black pepper.

Grill the bread on both sides and rub with the halved garlic clove. Top with the bean purée, then the mushroom mix. Serve with some salad leaves.

PER SERVING:
225 KCALS, 7G FAT, 1G SATURATED FAT, 32G CARBOHYDRATE, 0.36G SODIUM

stewed artichokes with spices and apricots and other things

A wonderfully spicy, nutritious vegetarian stew that is well worth the effort.

4 large globe artichokes
Juice of 1 lemon, lemon peel reserved
2 garlic cloves, finely sliced
10 black peppercorns
12 coriander seeds, toasted
½ teaspoon ground turmeric
¼ teaspoon cayenne pepper
½ teaspoon cumin seeds, toasted
2 onions, cut in eighths
2 bay leaves
50ml olive oil
Pinch of saffron strands, soaked in a little cold water
2 carrots, sliced
600ml vegetable stock
8 dried apricots, sliced
50g raisins
25g almonds, sliced
400g tinned chickpeas, drained and rinsed
225g baby spinach
2 tablespoons roughly chopped coriander leaves
4 tablespoons roughly chopped flat-leaf parsley

Serves 4

Trim the artichokes by peeling the stem until all woody matter has disappeared. Pull off all the tough outer leaves until you reach the pale green ones. Cut off about 2.5cm from the top of the artichoke. Cut the artichoke vertically into 4 and cut or pull out the choke. Rub all the cut surfaces with the lemon peel and place the artichoke quarters in a bowl of water. Add the lemon juice.

Using a mortar and pestle or coffee grinder, crush the garlic, peppercorns, coriander seeds, turmeric, cayenne and cumin seeds.

In a saucepan, cook the onions and bay leaves in the olive oil over a medium heat until they have softened but not coloured, this should take about 8 minutes. Add the spice mix and cook for a further 3 minutes.

Add the drained artichokes and the saffron with its soaking liquor and toss to combine. Add the carrots, half the vegetable stock, the apricots, raisins and almonds and simmer, covered for about 20 minutes, stirring from time to time. Add more stock as necessary.

When the artichokes are tender, add the chickpeas, spinach, coriander leaves and parsley and stir to combine. Cook until the spinach has wilted. Season with black pepper to taste.

Serve hot or cold with steamed couscous.

PER SERVING:
416 KCALS, 19G FAT, 2G SATURATED FAT, 46G CARBOHYDRATE, 0.52G SODIUM

stuffed peppers with brandade

A French dish, *brandade* is made by beating milk, olive oil and poached fish into a paste. Usually made with salt cod, it works equally well with fresh cod or haddock.

2 potatoes, cut into 2.5cm cubes
350g fresh cod
150ml semi-skimmed milk
2 garlic cloves, crushed
Juice of 1 lemon
2 tablespoons olive oil
50g ground almonds (optional)
Freshly ground black pepper
4 drained wood-roasted peppers
Lemon wedges, to serve

Serves 4

Cook the potatoes in water until soft. Mash and set aside.

Place the cod in a shallow frying pan, add the milk and bring to the boil. Remove from the heat and allow the cod to cool in the milk.

When the cod is cool enough to handle, remove from the milk and flake into a large bowl. Add the garlic, lemon juice, olive oil and almonds (if using) and combine well. Add the mashed potato to make a fairly thick paste. Season with black pepper to taste.

Stuff each pepper with the brandade paste and serve at room temperature, garnished with lemon wedges.

PER SERVING:
332 KCALS, 20G FAT, 3G SATURATED FAT, 19G CARBOHYDRATE, 1.28G SODIUM

tortino

This is similar to a *frittata* or *tortilla* in that the eggs hold the asparagus and spinach together to make a vegetarian 'cake' (colloquially, *tortino* means cake in Italian). Great for a light meal.

225g asparagus, cut into 2.5cm pieces
1 shallot, finely diced
10g unsalted butter
2 handfuls spinach, thick stems removed
1 teaspoon soft thyme leaves
5 large eggs, beaten
1 tablespoon skimmed milk
1 tablespoon grated Parmesan cheese
Freshly ground black pepper

Serves 4

Preheat the oven to 200°C/400°F/gas mark 6.

Blanch the asparagus in boiling water for 3 minutes, then refresh in cold water to arrest the cooking. Drain.

Pan-fry the shallot in the butter until softened but not coloured, then add the spinach and thyme leaves and cook until the leaves have wilted. Squeeze the liquid from the spinach and transfer the drained mix to a lightly buttered shallow baking dish. Place the asparagus over the spinach.

Beat the eggs, then combine with the milk and Parmesan. Season with black pepper and pour over the vegetables. Lift the vegetables slightly to allow the egg to cover the bottom of the dish.

Place in the oven and cook for about 15 minutes or until the eggs are set. This dish can be eaten hot or at room temperature.

PER SERVING:
162 KCALS, 12G FAT, 4G SATURATED FAT, 2G CARBOHYDRATE, 0.16G SODIUM

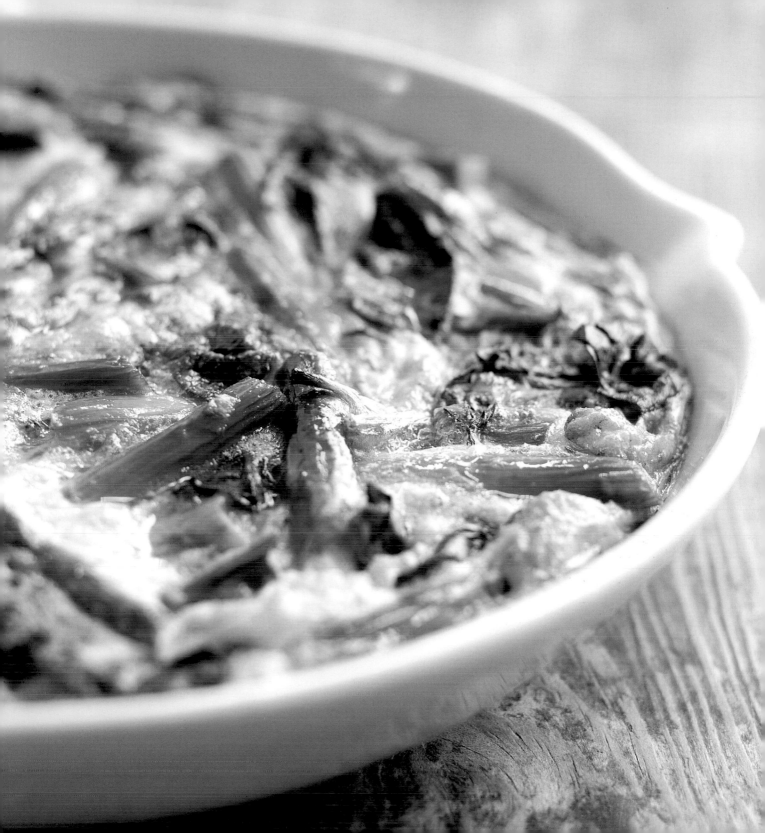

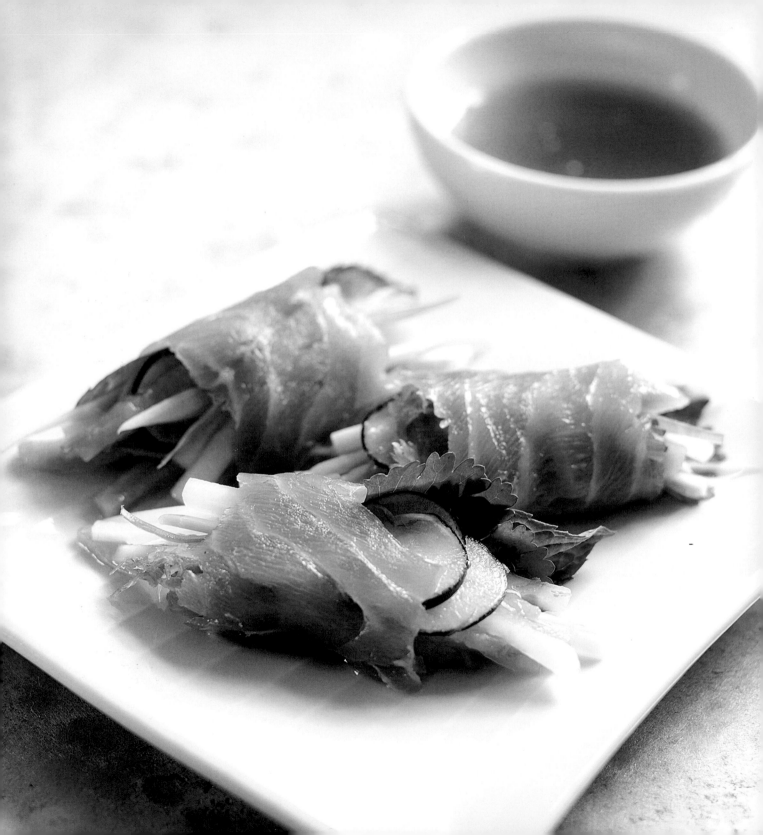

oriental smoked salmon rolls

Canapés, snacks, brunch – this is perfect for all kinds of occasions. Make sure that the fresh colours of the radish, paw-paw and cucumber peek out from the salmon rolls. Serve with some wholemeal toast.

1 green paw-paw or papaya, peeled and cut into thin matchsticks
½ cucumber, peeled and cut into thin matchsticks
8 radishes, thinly sliced
125ml rice wine vinegar
Juice and zest of 3 limes
1 tablespoon reduced-salt soy sauce
1 tablespoon runny honey
6 spring onions, finely shredded
350g smoked salmon, cut into long strips
48 mint leaves
48 coriander leaves

Makes 24 rolls

Combine the papaya, cucumber and radishes in a bowl.

Whisk together the rice wine vinegar, lime juice and zest, soy sauce and the honey, then pour over the papaya salad and allow to stand for 2 hours. Drain and fold in the spring onions.

Cut the smoked salmon in 7.5cm lengths. Place 2 leaves of each herb on the salmon, top with a little of the pickled vegetables and roll up tightly. Cover and refrigerate until ready to serve.

PER ROLL:
28 KCALS, 0.7G FAT, 0.1G SATURATED FAT, 2G CARBOHYDRATE, 0.3G SODIUM

salmon and haddock fishcakes

Everybody loves fishcakes and these are really good ones, great hot or cold. Serve with steamed vegetables and the Salsa Verde on page 62.

275g smoked haddock fillets
175g salmon fillets
600ml skimmed milk
1 onion, sliced
1 carrot, chopped
1 bay leaf
1 teaspoon black peppercorns
2 cloves
2 tablespoons olive oil
2 eggs

275g potatoes, cooked and mashed
2 teaspoons anchovy essence
2 eggs, hard-boiled, peeled and chopped
2 tablespoons chopped parsley
1 tablespoon chopped dill
Freshly ground black pepper
Plain flour
Fresh wholegrain breadcrumbs

Serves 4

Place the haddock and salmon in a large frying pan or roasting pan. Add enough milk to cover. Add one-third of the onion, the carrot, bay leaf, peppercorns and cloves. Bring to the boil and then simmer for 6 minutes. Set aside to cool slightly.

Dice the rest of the onion. Heat half of the olive oil in a pan and sweat the onion until softened, for about 6–8 minutes. Remove the fish from the milk and flake it, discarding any skin or bones. Strain the liquid and reserve. Beat 1 egg. Combine the haddock with the mashed potato, sweated onions, beaten egg and anchovy essence. Fold in the hard-boiled eggs, parsley and dill until well combined, but do not over-mix. Season with black pepper. If the mixture is too dry, mix in some of the strained fish liquid. Divide the mixture into four, and shape into patties.

Beat the remaining egg with a little water in a bowl. Season the flour and place on a plate. Place the breadcrumbs on another plate. Dip the patties in the flour, the egg and finally the breadcrumbs. Refrigerate for 2 hours.

Pan-fry the fishcakes in the remaining olive oil for 5 minutes on each side, and keep warm in the oven.

PER SERVING:
424 KCALS, 20G FAT, 5G SATURATED FAT, 28G CARBOHYDRATE, 0.91G SODIUM

stuffed sardines

This sardine dish has a hint of Moroccan influence, with its filling of nuts and currants. Sardines are a great-tasting oily fish, full of healthy omega-3 fatty acids.

1 red onion, very finely chopped
3 tablespoons olive oil
30g fresh wholegrain breadcrumbs
5 tablespoons currants, soaked in water for 15 minutes if very dry
3 tablespoons pine kernels
1 bunch flat-leaf parsley, chopped
5 tablespoons mixed lemon and orange juice
Freshly ground black pepper
Olive-oil spray (see page 17)
12 sardines, scaled, cleaned, flattened out and head and backbone removed
½ lemon, cut into 5mm thick slices
½ orange, cut into 5mm thick slices
12 fresh or 6 dried bay leaves, broken in half

Serves 4 as a starter (2 as a main course)

In a saucepan, sweat the onion in the olive oil. Add the breadcrumbs and cook for 2–3 minutes. Remove from the heat and add the currants, pine nuts and parsley. Pour in the citrus juices and stir. Season with black pepper and mix well. Allow to cool. Preheat the oven to 200°C/400°F/gas mark 6.

Lightly oil a baking dish with olive-oil spray. Fill each sardine with 1–2 teaspoons of filling. Roll each fish from head to tail. Pack the sardines tightly together in the dish with their tails sticking up in the same direction. Sprinkle them with the remaining filling. Place the orange and lemon slices and the bay leaves around the dish and tucked between the sardines. Bake for 10–15 minutes until golden. Serve warm or at room temperature.

PER SERVING:
489 KCALS, 29G FAT, 5G SATURATED FAT, 25G CARBOHYDRATE, 0.23G SODIUM

creamy sardines on toast

Sardines on toast never tasted so good. Tinned sardines also contain omega-3 fats and are a really versatile store-cupboard food. A great snack.

1 tablespoon olive oil
½ onion, finely diced
1 teaspoon soft thyme leaves
3 tablespoons wholemeal breadcrumbs
150ml low-fat yogurt
1 small tin sardines, drained and mashed
2 eggs, hard-boiled, peeled and chopped
Freshly ground black pepper
2 slices wholegrain bread

Serves 2

Heat the olive oil in a frying pan, add the onion and thyme and cook until the onion is soft but not brown. Add the remaining ingredients except the bread and warm through, stirring to combine. Season with black pepper to taste.

Preheat the grill. Toast the bread, then share the mixture equally between the slices. Pop under a hot grill until the mixture bubbles. Serve hot.

PER SERVING:
442 KCALS, 23G FAT, 5G SATURATED FAT, 29G CARBOHYDRATE, 0.73G SODIUM

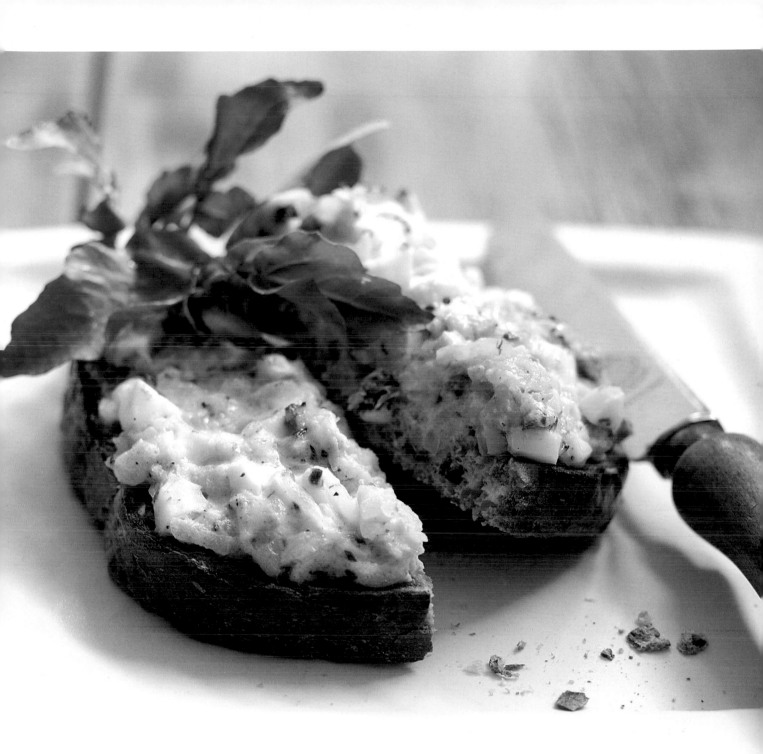

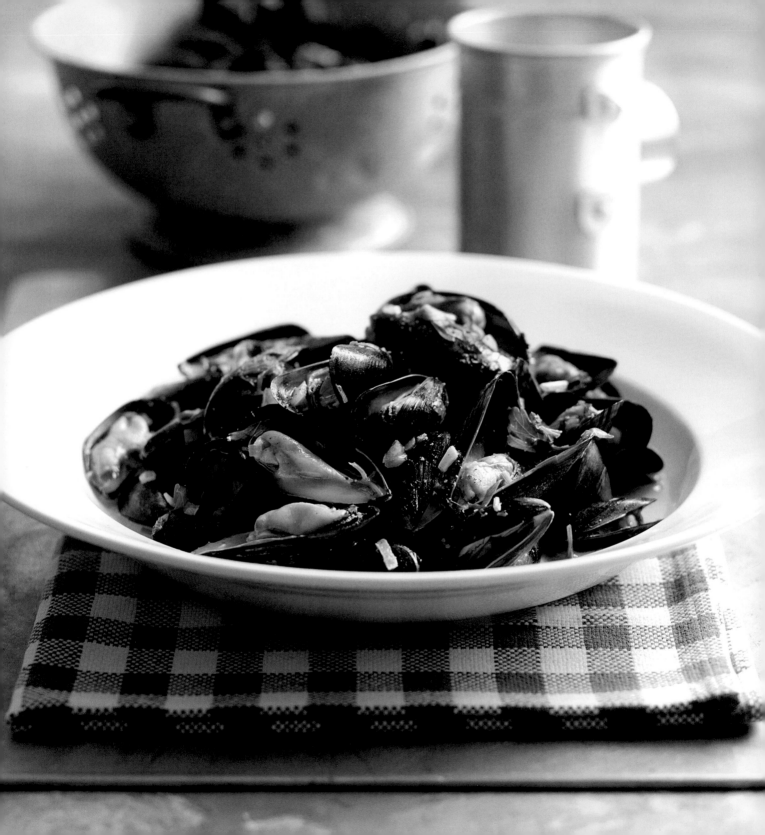

a bowl of steaming mussels

Mussels are such good value and this recipe is a variation on the traditional French dish, *Moules marinière*.

1 tablespoon olive oil
1 onion, finely diced
4 tinned anchovy fillets, drained, rinsed and chopped
4 large garlic cloves, chopped
1 red chilli, chopped
1 glass white wine
150ml fish stock
1kg mussels, cleaned
4 tablespoons finely chopped parsley
Freshly ground black pepper

Serves 4 as a starter (2 as a main course)

Heat the olive oil in a large saucepan over a medium heat. Add the onion, anchovies, garlic and chilli and cook until the onion is soft but not brown. Add the wine and the stock and bring to the boil. Simmer for 5 minutes, then add the mussels and cover. Increase the heat and cook for approximately 5 minutes, shaking the pan from time to time.

Remove the mussels with a slotted spoon to warm bowls, discarding any that have not opened.

Boil the remaining liquid for a further 2 minutes, then add the parsley and season with ground black pepper. Pour over the mussels and serve with crusty wholegrain bread.

PER SERVING:
130 KCALS, 5G FAT, 1G SATURATED FAT, 6G CARBOHYDRATE, 0.39G SODIUM

sardines with tomatoes and red onion

Another great sardine recipe, this makes a delicious light lunch or supper, simple to prepare with ingredients that you will probably have in your cupboard. Serve with seeded bread or toast.

500g fresh plum tomatoes, sliced
½ red onion, finely sliced
2 tins of sardines, drained and rinsed
3 pinches of dried oregano
Pinch of dried red chilli flakes
Freshly ground black pepper
Balsamic vinegar, to taste
Fresh marjoram leaves
Handful of black olives

Serves 4

Arrange the tomato slices on a serving plate so that they overlap. Scatter with red onion slices. Arrange the sardines carefully over the tomatoes. Sprinkle the sardines with oregano, chilli flakes and freshly ground black pepper.

Drizzle a little balsamic vinegar over the plate. Garnish with some fresh marjoram leaves and black olives. Serve at room temperature.

PER SERVING:
192 KCALS, 11G FAT, 2G SATURATED FAT, 6G CARBOHYDRATE, 0.47G SODIUM

tuna kebabs with pickled lemon and mint

Great for a barbecue, these kebabs are both tasty and nutritious. Tuna and tomatoes are Mediterranean 'musts', especially when combined with sunshine! Delicious with pitta bread and salad.

4 pickled lemons
1 bunch mint, leaves only
4 garlic cloves, roughly chopped
½ teaspoon dried red chilli flakes
1 tablespoon olive oil
1kg tuna loin, cut into 16 even-sized cubes
12 bay leaves
12 cherry tomatoes

Serves 4

Cut the pickled lemons in half, scoop out the flesh and discard. Cut the rinds of 3 of the lemons into 12 pieces of roughly even size. Place the rind of the fourth lemon in a food processor with the mint, garlic, chilli flakes, oil and 2 tablespoons of water and pulse until smooth. Spoon into a bowl, then add the tuna pieces and marinate for 20 minutes.

Slide 1 piece of tuna on to a bamboo skewer that has been soaked in water. Follow the tuna with 1 bay leaf, 1 tomato and 1 piece of lemon rind. Do this three more times, finishing the kebab with a piece of tuna. Prepare three more skewers in this way.

Preheat the grill to its highest setting or heat a large frying pan or griddle pan. Char-grill the skewers for 1 minute on each side until they are medium rare, or as you like them. Serve with a leaf salad.

PER SERVING:
393 KCALS, 15G FAT, 4G SATURATED FAT, 5G CARBOHYDRATE, 0.52G SODIUM

anchovy toasts

An unusual dish, but it's worth being a little avant-garde for these delicious flavours. Anchovies are usually bought tinned, but fresh anchovies are a delicacy in Portugal, Spain and Turkey.

4 dried figs, roughly chopped
1 tablespoon Pernod
4 tablespoons green tea
50g whole almonds, toasted
25g macadamia nuts
4 spring onions, roughly chopped
2 garlic cloves, roughly chopped
1 teaspoon tarragon leaves
1 teaspoon dill leaves
1 teaspoon flat-leaf parsley
2 sun-dried tomatoes, drained
3 cherry peppers, seeded
Juice and zest of 2 limes
1 tablespoon olive oil
4 slices wholegrain bread, toasted
8 tinned anchovy fillets, drained, rinsed and sliced in half lengthways

Serves 4 (2 as a main course)

Preheat the oven to 200°C/400°F/gas mark 6.

Soak the figs in the Pernod and tea for 2 hours. Combine the figs with the remaining ingredients except the toast and anchovies.

Spread the fig mixture on the toast and cook in the oven for 10 minutes. Cut each slice into 2 pieces and top with the anchovy fillets. Eat while hot.

PER SERVING:
315 KCALS, 18G FAT, 2G SATURATED FAT, 30G CARBOHYDRATE, 0.5G SODIUM

trout in a red pepper blanket

Trout is such an underrated fish, but it is excellent value, great tasting and high in omega-3. Together with red peppers and garlic, this is an unbeatable combination.

3 red peppers, seeded and quartered
50g pine kernels, toasted
50g fresh breadcrumbs
3 garlic cloves, finely chopped
Olive-oil spray (see page 17)
Freshly ground black pepper
4 'spatchcocked' trout (ask your fishmonger to open and fillet the trout, removing the head and tail)

Serves 4

Char the peppers in the oven or over a gas flame until the skin is blackened. Place the peppers in a paper bag and seal. Allow the peppers to steam in their own heat for 15 minutes, then remove and peel. Place in a food processor with their juice and blend.

Add the pine kernels, breadcrumbs and garlic and blend again to a smooth purée. With the food processor running, add the olive oil in a thin stream. Season with black pepper to taste.

Rub the trout on both sides with the red pepper purée. Refrigerate for 30 minutes.

Heat a ridged griddle plate, large frying pan or barbecue until very hot. Lightly spray the surface with olive oil and cook the trout, flesh-side down, for 3 minutes. Turn the fish carefully and cook for a further 3 minutes.

Transfer to a serving platter and serve with noodles, rice or new potatoes.

PER SERVING:
369 KCALS, 16G FAT, 3G SATURATED FAT, 18G CARBOHYDRATE, 0.2G SODIUM

chilli-corn crabcakes

Crabcakes are an all-time favourite of mine and these can be made the day before and stored in the fridge. White crab meat comes from the claw, the brown meat from the body. Serve with a green salad.

450g white crab meat, picked over
225g brown crab meat
1 chilli, finely diced
1 onion, finely diced
½ red pepper, seeded and finely diced
2 celery sticks, finely diced
200g tinned sweetcorn, drained
2 teaspoons chopped dill
150ml low-fat Greek yogurt
1 teaspoon mustard powder
2 eggs, lightly beaten
50g fresh wholemeal breadcrumbs
3 tablespoons rapeseed oil
Freshly ground black pepper

Serves 6

In a large bowl, mix together the white and brown crab meat, chilli, onion, red pepper, celery, sweetcorn and dill.

Combine the yogurt, mustard powder and eggs in another bowl and then slowly add half the oil. Add the crab mixture and mix well. Fold in a third of the breadcrumbs, or as much as you need to firm the mixture, and season to taste with black pepper. Refrigerate for 2 hours ideally.

Make the mixture into 6 large or 12 small patties. Coat each one in the remaining breadcrumbs. These cakes can be made well ahead of when they are needed; at this point put them in the fridge to dry out overnight.

Heat the remaining oil in a large pan over a medium heat, and cook the cakes for 3 minutes on each side. Serve hot.

PER SERVING:
306 KCALS, 16G FAT, 3G SATURATED FAT, 14G CARBOHYDRATE, 0.64G SODIUM

chicken liver pâté

The easiest pâté I know, this takes just minutes to prepare. Eat hot or cold, with pickles, Melba toast or crusty wholegrain bread, for a great snack or lunch.

Rapeseed-oil spray (see page 17)
225g chicken livers, cleaned
300ml skimmed milk
3 egg yolks
1 shallot, finely diced
1 garlic clove, finely diced
1 teaspoon soft thyme leaves
Freshly ground black pepper
25g fresh breadcrumbs

Serves 4

Preheat the oven to 160°C/325°F/gas mark 3.

Lightly spray 4 small moulds or ramekins with oil.

Put the livers, milk, egg yolks, shallot, garlic and thyme in a food processor and blend until smooth. Season with black pepper.

Pass through a fine sieve and then fold in the breadcrumbs.

Spoon the mixture into the moulds and then place in a roasting tray. Add hot water to the tray until it comes three-quarters of way up the sides of the moulds. Cook in the oven until the pâté has set, this should take about 20 minutes.

PER SERVING:
150 KCALS, 6G FAT, 2G SATURATED FAT, 9G CARBOHYDRATE, 0.14G SODIUM

chicken stir-fry with black beans

Chinese food offers lots of flavours, but very little fat. In fact, along with the Mediterranean diet, it is one we could learn a few tips from.

1 egg white
3 teaspoons cornflour
2 skinless chicken breasts, cut into thin strips
½ tablespoon groundnut oil
2 garlic cloves, finely chopped
2.5cm fresh root ginger, peeled and grated
Pinch of dried red chilli flakes
1 tablespoon Chinese black beans, finely chopped
1 carrot, sliced on the diagonal
½ red pepper, seeded and cut into diamonds
½ yellow pepper, seeded and cut into diamonds
125ml chicken stock
1 tablespoon reduced-salt dark soy sauce
2 tablespoons rice wine vinegar
Pinch of sugar
75g sugar-snap peas
4 spring onions, sliced on the diagonal

Serves 2

Lightly beat the egg white in a non-metallic bowl with half the cornflour. Add the chicken, cover with clingfilm and chill for 30 minutes (this is called velveting).

Place 300ml water in a pan and bring to the boil. Stir the chicken and then remove from the bowl with a slotted spoon. Remove the pan from the heat and add the chicken, stirring to prevent it from sticking together, then return to the heat and cook for 1½ minutes or until the chicken is white and just tender. Drain on kitchen paper.

Heat a wok and swirl in the oil. Add the garlic, ginger, chilli flakes and black beans and stir-fry for 15 seconds, then add the carrot and stir-fry for 1 minute. Stir in the cooked chicken and the peppers. Pour in the stock, then add the soy sauce, vinegar and sugar, stirring to combine.

Increase the heat and bring to the boil, then reduce to a simmer. Add the sugar-snap peas and spring onions and cook for 2 minutes. Mix the remaining cornflour with 1 tablespoon water and stir into the wok. Cook for a minute or so until the sauce clears and thickens. Serve at once with steamed rice.

PER SERVING:
289 KCALS, 5G FAT, 1G SATURATED FAT, 22G CARBOHYDRATE, 0.95G SODIUM

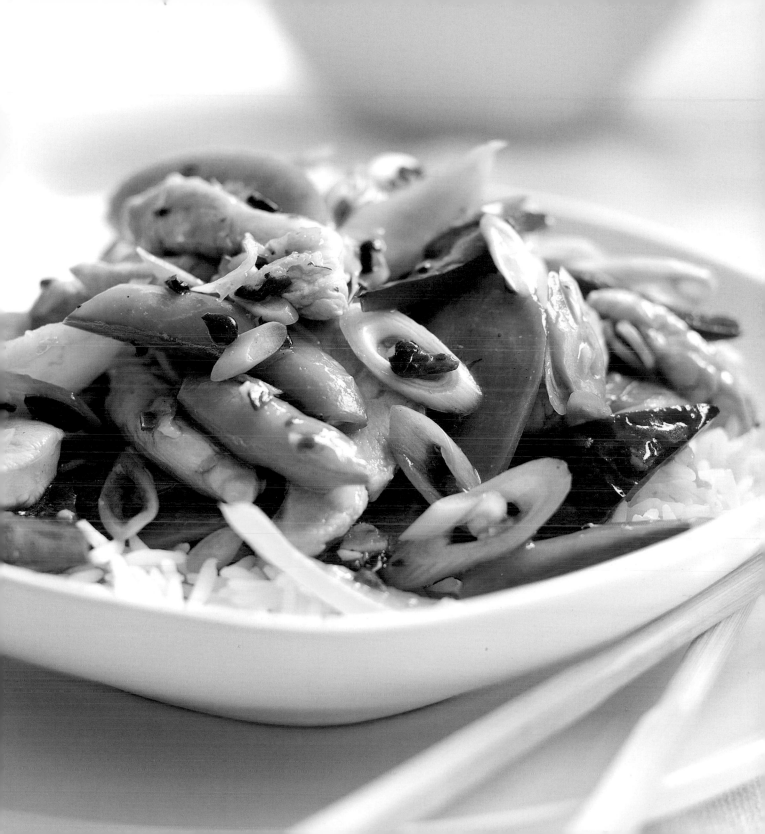

hot chilli chicken fajitas

Mexico in its most popular foodie form. The cool flavours of the salsa take the edge off the hot chicken marinade and it needs no further accompaniment. Cook on the barbecue or a griddle pan.

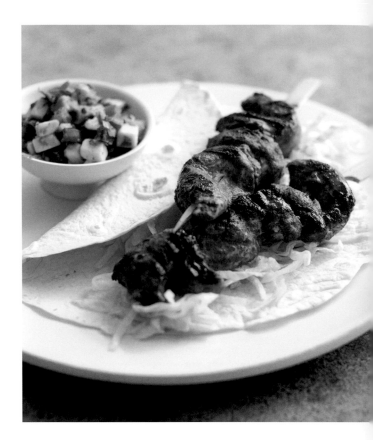

1 tablespoon chilli oil
1 tablespoon hot chilli powder
1 tablespoon paprika
Pinch of caster sugar
Grated zest and juice of 1 lime
2 skinless chicken breast fillets
4 soft flour tortillas
¼ small iceberg lettuce, shredded
75ml low-fat yogurt

For the tomato and avocado salsa
2 large tomatoes, seeded and finely diced
1 red chilli, seeded and finely chopped
Juice of 1 lime
½ small red onion, finely chopped
1 ripe avocado, peeled, stoned and finely diced
1 tablespoon olive oil
8 tablespoons roughly chopped coriander leaves
Freshly ground black pepper

Serves 4

Soak eight 15cm bamboo skewers in water overnight.

Mix together the chilli oil, chilli powder, paprika, sugar and the lime zest and juice in a shallow non-metallic dish.

Cut each chicken breast lengthways into 6 strips. Add to the chilli mixture and stir until well coated, then cover with clingfilm and leave to marinate in the fridge for 1–2 hours.

To make the tomato and avocado salsa, place all the ingredients into a large bowl and stir gently to combine. Season with black pepper to taste and spoon into a serving bowl. Cover with clingfilm and set aside to allow the flavours to develop, but don't make this too far in advance otherwise the avocado may blacken.

Heat a griddle pan or a barbecue. Thread 3 pieces of chicken on to each soaked bamboo skewer and place on the griddle pan or barbecue. Cook for 3–4 minutes on each side or until the chicken is cooked through and lightly charred.

Heat a frying or griddle pan. Add a tortilla and heat for 30 seconds, or until soft and pliable, turning once. Repeat with the remaining tortillas and stack up on a warmed plate. Place the chicken skewers on a serving platter and hand around the tomato and avocado salsa, warmed tortillas, lettuce and yogurt, allowing each person to assemble the fajitas themselves.

PER SERVING:
392 KCALS, 15G FAT, 2G SATURATED FAT, 42G CARBOHYDRATE, 0.27G SODIUM

souvlakia

Memories of Greek holidays, hot sun, white sands and warm seas. This Mediterranean staple makes a simple but filling meal, great also for packed lunches and picnics.

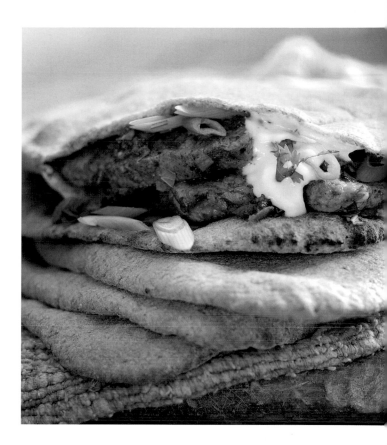

450g lamb fillets, cut into 1cm slices
1 onion, grated
6 garlic cloves, mashed to a paste with a little salt
2 teaspoons freshly ground black pepper
2 teaspoons ground cumin
1 teaspoon cayenne pepper
4 tablespoons olive oil
4 wholemeal pitta breads
Juice of 1 lemon
8 tablespoons low-fat yogurt
1 teaspoon chopped mint leaves
1 teaspoon chopped coriander leaves
6 spring onions, sliced

Serves 4

Toss the lamb with the onion, garlic, black pepper, cumin, cayenne pepper and 1 tablespoon olive oil. Allow to marinate for as long as possible and at least 1 hour.

Heat the remaining olive oil in a heavy-based saucepan and cook the lamb for 2 minutes on each side. Warm the pitta breads, and cut the edges to form a pocket. Stuff the lamb into the pocket and dribble with the lemon juice, yogurt, fresh herbs and spring onions.

PER SERVING:
478 KCALS, 23G FAT, 7G SATURATED FAT, 38G CARBOHYDRATE, 0.5G SODIUM

linguine with fiery prawns

Add a little fire to your belly. The tomato sauce has a surprising kick to it that will wake up your appetite and warm your mouth.

3 tablespoons olive oil
2 teaspoons dried red chilli flakes or dried crushed chillies
1 teaspoon chopped thyme
400g tinned chopped tomatoes
5 garlic cloves, finely chopped
250g baby spinach
Freshly ground black pepper
450g raw large prawns, shelled and split lengthways
225g dried wholemeal linguine
2 tablespoons chopped flat-leaf parsley

Serves 4

Heat half the oil in a frying-pan over a medium heat. Add the chilli flakes and cook for 1 minute. Add the thyme, tomatoes and half the garlic, and stir well to combine. Cook for about 15 minutes, until the sauce has reduced and thickened. Fold in the spinach leaves and cook for 3 minutes. Season with black pepper to taste.

In a separate pan, heat the remaining oil with the remaining garlic. When the garlic begins to colour, add the prawns and cook until just pink, this should take about 2 minutes. Keep warm.

Meanwhile, cook the linguine in plenty of boiling water until al dente. Drain and place in a warm shallow serving dish.

Add the prawns, tomato sauce and parsley to the linguine and combine thoroughly. Serve immediately.

PER SERVING:
385 KCALS, 11G FAT, 2G SATURATED FAT, 43G CARBOHYDRATE, 0.47G SODIUM

fettuccine with purple sprouting broccoli

Purple sprouting broccoli, a springtime speciality knocks the spots off other broccoli. Broccoli is also a superveg, one of the most nutritious around.

1 onion, finely diced
1 garlic clove, finely chopped
4 tinned anchovy fillets, drained, rinsed and finely chopped
2 teaspoons tinned capers, drained, rinsed and chopped
1 teaspoon rosemary leaves
1 tablespoon chopped flat-leaf parsley
1 tablespoon olive oil
350g purple sprouting broccoli, cut into 5cm pieces
450g fresh fettuccine
Juice of ½ lemon
Freshly ground black pepper
Parmesan cheese shavings

Serves 4

In a saucepan, cook the first 6 ingredients in the olive oil, until the onions have softened without colouring.

Meanwhile, boil the broccoli in plenty of boiling water for 2 minutes, add the fettuccine and cook for a further 3 minutes. When the pasta is cooked and the broccoli has broken up slightly, remove and drain.

Place the pasta and broccoli in a bowl and combine with the hot dressing. Add the lemon juice and season with black pepper to taste. Serve sprinkled with shavings of Parmesan.

PER SERVING:
387 KCALS, 7G FAT, 1G SATURATED FAT, 68G CARBOHYDRATE, 0.22G SODIUM

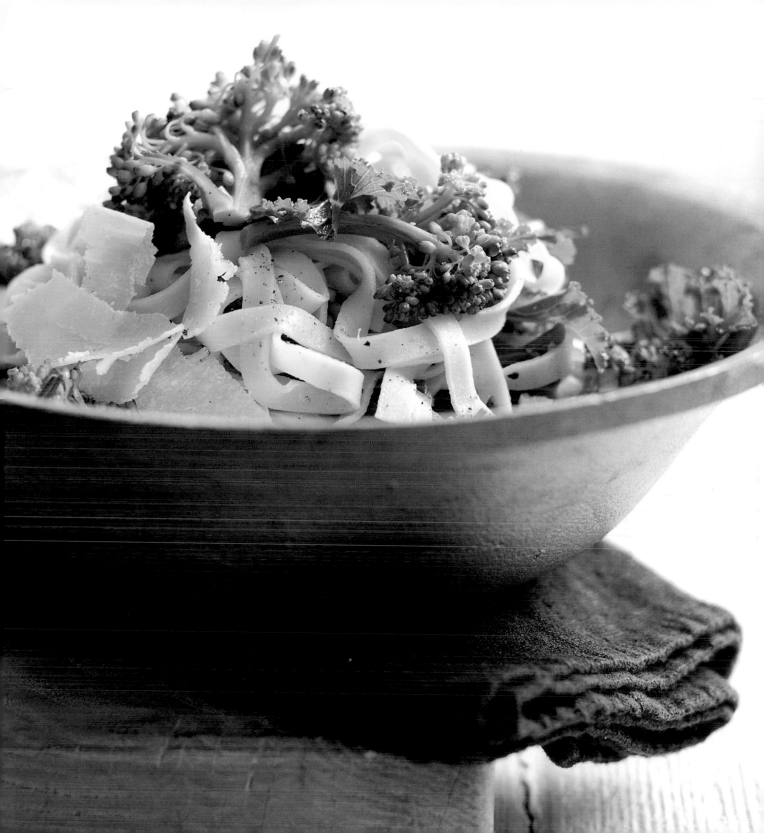

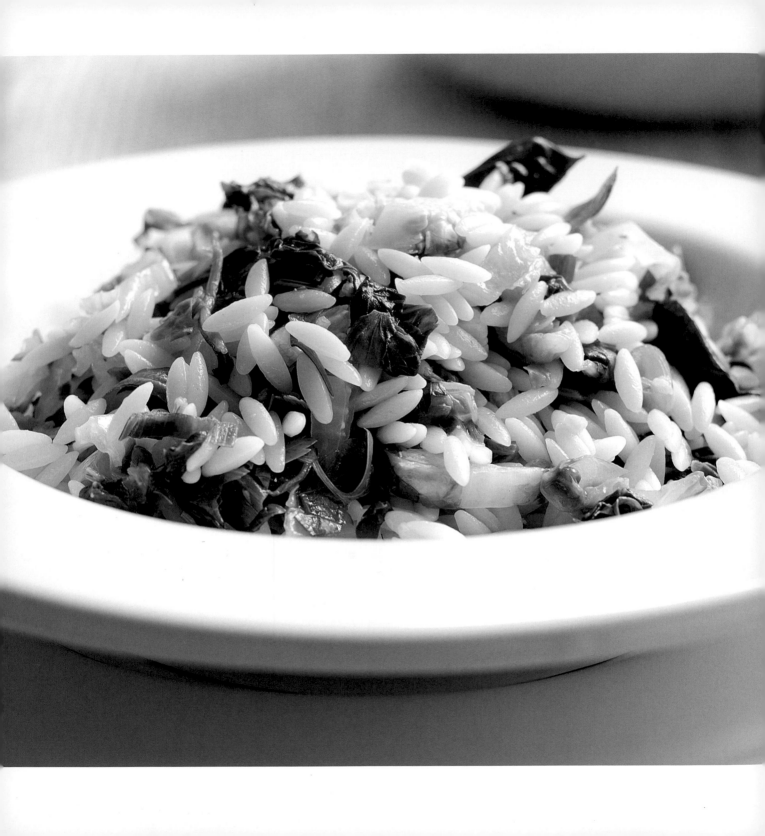

green pasta

The herbs and spinach provide this pasta with a little extra goodness. Quick and simple, this is also low in fat, but immensely satisfying. Great for a light lunch or dinner.

350g orsi or risoni
   (rice-shaped pasta)
2 tablespoons olive oil
2 garlic cloves, finely chopped
Pinch of dried chilli flakes
2 handfuls of spinach, chopped
6 spring onions, finely sliced
2 Little Gem lettuces, shredded
Handful flat-leaf parsley leaves, roughly chopped
12 basil leaves, ripped
Juice of 1 lemon

Serves 6

Cook the pasta in a large saucepan of boiling water, then drain and return to the saucepan.

Meanwhile, heat the olive oil in a large wok, add the garlic and chilli flakes and cook for 1 minute. Add the spinach and, using a pair of tongs, keep turning the spinach over until it has wilted, this should take about 3 minutes. Add the remaining ingredients and cook for a further 2 minutes. Season with black pepper to taste.

Add the greens to the pasta and toss to combine, then serve immediately.

PER SERVING:
247 KCALS, 5G FAT, 1G SATURATED FAT, 45G CARBOHYDRATE, 0.02G SODIUM

black olive dip

Another Mediterranean must, this is great served with raw vegetables or spread on wholegrain toast. A very moreish dip that will keep you going until you run out of vegetables.

225g black olives, pitted
2 tablespoons olive oil
2 garlic cloves, finely chopped
Pinch of dried red chilli flakes

½ teaspoon ground black pepper
1 tablespoon tinned capers, drained
   and rinsed
Grated zest and juice of
   1 lemon
1 tablespoon chopped parsley

Serves 8

Blend all the ingredients in a food processor and blitz until smooth – unless you prefer to leave it slightly chunky.

PER SERVING:
57 KCALS, 6G FAT, 1G SATURATED FAT, 1G CARBOHYDRATE, 0.68G SODIUM

fiery marinated olives

350g black and/or green
   olives, pitted, rinsed and dried
1 teaspoon harissa or chilli sauce
4 tablespoons lemon juice

1 heaped tablespoon pickled lemon
   rind, chopped (optional)
225ml olive oil
Finely pared zest of 1 orange
   (unwaxed, if possible)
2 garlic cloves, quartered

Fills a 600ml kilner jar

Place all the ingredients in a non-metallic bowl and stir until well combined. Transfer to a sterilised kilner jar with a tight-fitting lid or simply leave in the bowl and cover tightly with clingfilm. Set aside for 4 days or up to 2 weeks before eating (after that the garlic could become rancid).

Drain the oil and lay the olives on kitchen paper to remove any excess before serving. Be warned – they are very potent.

PER 25G:
57 KCALS, 6.2G FAT, 0.9G SATURATED FAT, 0G CARBOHYDRATE, 0.49G SODIUM

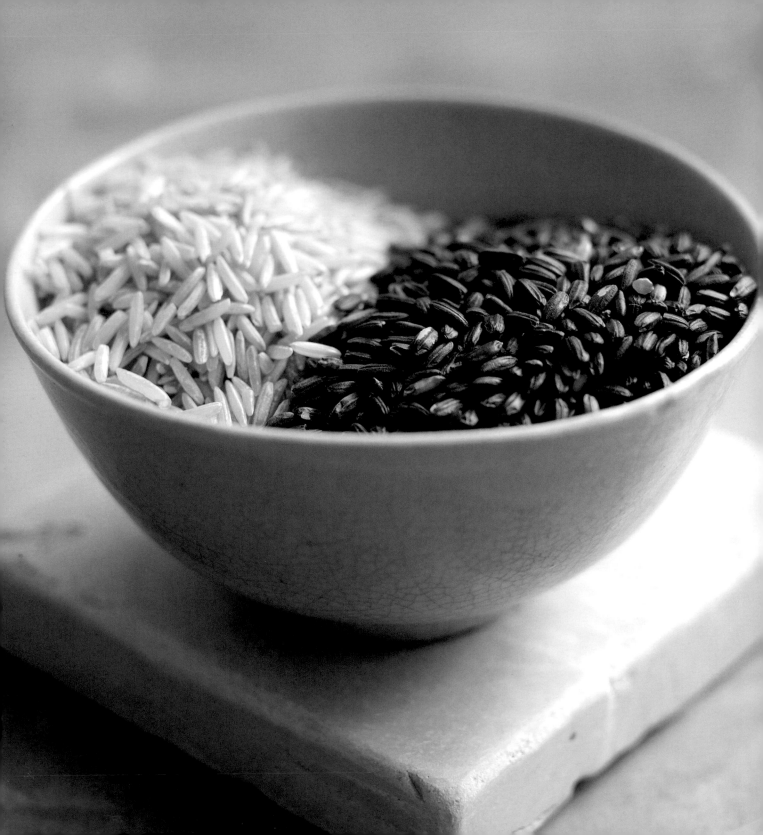

4

main courses

saffron pea pilaff

A pilaff is a Middle Eastern rice dish, often cooked with meat or vegetables. In a pilaff the grains of rice should remain as separate as possible, so the rice is rinsed thoroughly first. Serve with a salad.

225g brown rice
1 tablespoon olive oil
25g margarine
25g flaked almonds
8 walnut halves, roughly chopped
25g raisins
8 dried apricots, diced
4 cloves
2 cardamom pods
2.5cm cinnamon stick
½ teaspoon saffron strands, soaked in a little warm water
4 spring onions, thinly sliced
Freshly ground black pepper
1 litre vegetable or chicken stock
375g podded peas (fresh or frozen)
3 tablespoons chopped coriander

Serves 4

Rinse the rice with cold water, then drain and set aside.

Heat the olive oil and margarine in a large heavy-based pan that has a tight-fitting lid. Add the almonds, walnuts, raisins and apricots and cook for about 5 minutes until the nuts are golden brown and the raisins are plumped up, stirring occasionally and taking care that nothing burns. Remove the fruit and nuts with a slotted spoon and set aside.

Add the cloves, cardamom pods and cinnamon stick to the pan. Cook gently for a minute or two until they become aromatic, stirring continuously. Add the drained rice to the pan and cook for 2 minutes, stirring to ensure all the rice grains are coated, then stir in the saffron mixture, the spring onions and ½ teaspoon pepper. Pour in the stock, bring to the boil, then reduce the heat, cover and simmer for 45 minutes or until the rice is fluffed up and completely tender. Add more stock as necessary, but remember it should end up quite dry.

When the pilaff has nearly finished cooking, place the peas in a pan of boiling water and simmer for 2–3 minutes until tender, then drain. Remove the pilaff from the heat and add the peas, fruit and nut mixture and the coriander. Gently fold in using a large metal spoon until well combined. Season with black pepper to taste and serve hot.

PER SERVING:
492 KCALS, 19G FAT, 3G SATURATED FAT, 70G CARBOHYDRATE, 0.38G SODIUM

pumpkin risotto with leek and yogurt

Risottos are usually quite high in fat as they are generally made with cream, butter and cheese. This version uses less cheese and low-fat yogurt. Serve with a salad.

2 tablespoons olive oil
350g pumpkin, peeled and cut into 2.5cm dice
2 leeks, sliced
1 tablespoon chopped sage
Freshly ground black pepper
2 onions, finely chopped
1 heaped teaspoon thyme leaves
1 fresh bay leaf
225g arborio (risotto) rice
1 glass dry white wine
1 litre vegetable stock, boiling
25g Parmesan cheese, grated
85g low-fat Greek yogurt
2 tablespoons flat-leaf parsley, chopped

Serves 4

Heat half of the oil in a large sauté pan, add the pumpkin and cook over a fairly high heat for about 5 minutes until lightly caramelised, tossing occasionally. Reduce the heat, add the leeks and sage, and cook over a gentle heat, stirring occasionally, for another 2–3 minutes until softened but not coloured and the pumpkin is completely tender when pierced with the tip of a sharp knife. Season with black pepper, tip into a bowl and set aside.

Add the remaining oil to the pumpkin pan, then tip in the onions, thyme and bay leaf and cook for a few minutes until softened but not coloured, stirring occasionally.

Add the rice to the onion mixture and continue to cook for another minute, stirring to ensure that all the grains are well coated. Pour in the wine and allow to bubble down, stirring until it is completely absorbed.

Begin to add the boiling stock a ladle at a time, stirring frequently. Allow each addition to be almost completely absorbed before adding the next. After approximately 20 minutes, add the pumpkin mixture, the Parmesan, yogurt and parsley, and stir energetically to combine.

Season with black pepper to taste and serve immediately with a big bowl of salad leaves.

PER SERVING:
359 KCALS, 10G FAT, 3G SATURATED FAT, 54G CARBOHYDRATE, 0.41G SODIUM

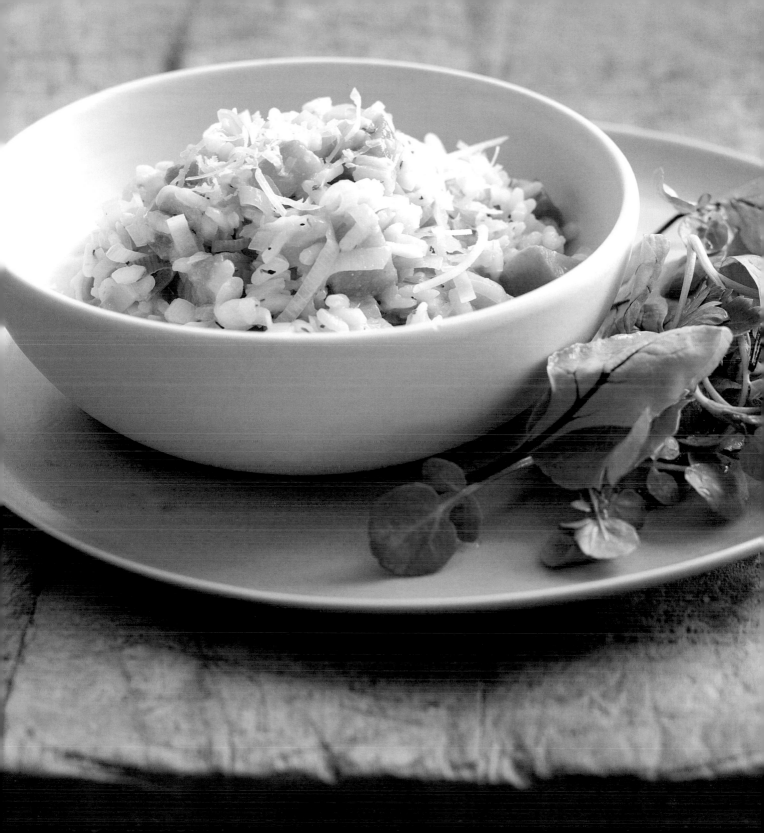

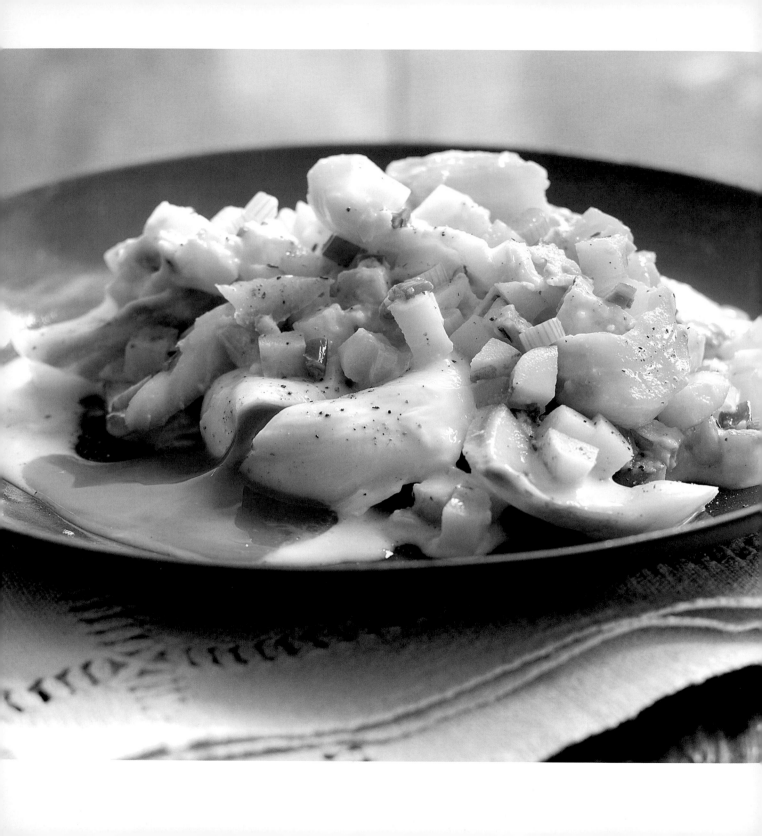

smoked haddock and potato 'risotto'

Smoked food tends to be high in salt, so keep the rest of your day's salt intake as low as possible. Children, pregnant women and the elderly should not eat undercooked eggs. Serve with a leaf salad.

600ml semi-skimmed milk
1 onion, halved
1 fresh bay leaf
225g undyed smoked haddock
1 garlic clove, finely chopped
2 spring onions, finely sliced
1 sprig thyme

1 tablespoon olive oil
225g unpeeled new
    potatoes, diced
25g Parmesan cheese,
    grated
2 tablespoons low-fat Greek
    yogurt
Freshly ground black pepper
2 soft poached eggs

Serves 2

Heat the milk in a saucepan with the onion and bay leaf. Remove from the heat and allow to infuse for 15 minutes. Return to the heat. When simmering, add the fish and cook for 8 minutes. Remove the fish and set aside, then strain the cooking liquid.

Cook the garlic, spring onions and thyme in the olive oil for 5 minutes, then add the potatoes and cooking milk and cook until the potatoes are tender, this should take about 12 minutes.

Flake the smoked haddock, discarding any skin or bones and fold into the potato mix. Fold in the Parmesan and yogurt, then season with black pepper to taste.

Fill a deep pan with water and bring to the boil, the water should be at least 12cm deep. Add 1½ tablespoons vinegar for every 1 litre of water. Crack each egg into a coffee cup and slide the egg into the water at the exact point where it has a rolling boil. After 2-3 minutes of cooking lift the eggs with a slotted spoon and lower them into iced water.

Warm through the poached eggs and place one on each warm plate. Top with the smoked haddock 'risotto'.

PER SERVING:
506 KCALS, 22G FAT, 9G SATURATED FAT, 35G CARBOHYDRATE, 1.25G SODIUM

prawn and saffron risotto

A more traditional risotto than the smoked haddock and potato version (left), this is a creamy emulsion of flavour and texture, rich and very delicious. Serve with a leaf salad.

1.2 litres fish stock
3 tablespoons olive oil
1 onion, finely diced
3 garlic cloves, finely diced
2 red chillies, finely diced
½ teaspoon chopped thyme
2 fresh bay leaves

375g Arborio (risotto) rice
2 tablespoons dry vermouth
2 pinches of saffron strands, soaked
    in 2 tablespoons cold water
36 raw, shelled prawns
20 basil leaves, torn
2 tablespoons pesto
2 tablespoons low-fat Greek yogurt
Freshly ground black pepper

Serves 4

Bring the fish stock to the boil in a large saucepan and keep at a simmer.

Heat another large saucepan and add the olive oil. Stir in the onion, garlic, chillies, thyme and bay leaves, and cook until the onion is soft but without colour. Add the rice and cook for 3 minutes.

Add the vermouth and stir until the liquid is almost completely absorbed. Add the saffron with its soaking liquid and a ladle of hot fish stock. Before adding further stock, allow the liquid to be absorbed. Stir the rice frequently. Continue to add hot stock, a ladleful at a time, allowing each addition to be absorbed before you add the next. The idea is to keep the rice creamy and thick like a sauce. As you add more stock, the rice will release its starches and start to puff up. After about 20 minutes, nibble on a grain of rice to see whether it is cooked; there should still be a little bite to it.

When the risotto is ready it will have a creamy texture, with the grains of rice still separate. Add the prawns and basil, stirring as you cook for a further 2 minutes. Fold in the pesto, yogurt and seasoning. Serve immediately

PER SERVING:
531 KCALS, 12G FAT, 2G SATURATED FAT, 78G CARBOHYDRATE, 0.64G SODIUM

bay-scented salmon on roasted vegetables

Salmon is a fantastic fish, full of omega-3 fats, but farmed salmon can be less flavoursome than wild. Either way, this dish provides all the taste it needs.

3 small carrots, halved
2 small parsnips, halved
6 large shallots
½ small butternut squash, peeled, seeded and cut into wedges
2 garlic cloves, crushed
1 red chilli, seeded and finely chopped

1 teaspoon thyme leaves
1 tablespoon olive oil
1 teaspoon freshly ground black pepper
Olive-oil spray (see page 17)
16 fresh bay leaves
4 x 175g salmon steaks
Juice and zest of 1 lime
3 tablespoons chopped chervil

Serves 4

Place half the bay leaves on a plate, top with the salmon steaks and the remaining bay leaves and season with ground black pepper. Cover with clingfilm and refrigerate for 1 hour. Preheat the oven to 190°C/375°F/gas mark 5.

Place the carrots, parsnips, whole shallots and the squash in a pan of boiling water and blanch for 2–3 minutes, then refresh under cold running water to retain their colour.

Toss together the cooked vegetables, garlic, chilli and thyme with the olive oil and place in a preheated baking dish. Pop in the oven and roast for 45 minutes or until the vegetables are tender and golden, turning from time to time. Season with black pepper.

About 10 minutes before the vegetables are ready, lightly spray a baking tray with olive oil. Place the bay leaves and the salmon on top, spray the salmon with a little oil and season with black pepper. Grill for 5 minutes on each side.

Serve the salmon on a bed of the roasted vegetables, squeeze a little lime juice over the salmon, sprinkle with the lime zest and chervil and serve with lime wedges.

PER SERVING:
422 KCALS, 23G FAT, 4G SATURATED FAT, 17G CARBOHYDRATE, 0.1G SODIUM

salmon with pea and watercress purée

Steaming is one of the best ways to cook as the food retains more nutrients, but it is perceived as boring. This should change your mind. Most of the fat here is unsaturated. Serve with steamed new potatoes.

Olive-oil spray (see page 17)
4 spring onions, thinly sliced
175g podded peas (fresh or frozen)
300ml vegetable stock
85g watercress
2 tablespoons low-fat Greek yogurt
Freshly ground black pepper
2 x 175g salmon steaks
Lemon wedges

Serves 2

Heat a non-stick sauté pan and lightly spray with oil. Add the spring onions and cook for a few minutes until softened, stirring occasionally. Add the peas and stock to the pan, stirring to combine. Cover with a circle of greaseproof paper and allow to sweat for 2-3 minutes.

Remove the paper and add the watercress, reserving a little for the garnish, then allow to cook for a further 2 minutes or until all the liquid has evaporated. Place in a food processor with the yogurt and blend until nearly smooth – you still want a little texture. Season with black pepper to taste. Set aside.

Season the salmon fillets with black pepper and steam for 6 minutes; alternatively wrap them in foil and place in a preheated oven at 200°C/400°F/gas mark 6 for 8 minutes.

Place the salmon on the pea purée and garnish with the lemon wedges and reserved watercress.

PER SERVING:
431 KCALS, 23G FAT, 5G SATURATED FAT, 13G CARBOHYDRATE, 0.31G SODIUM

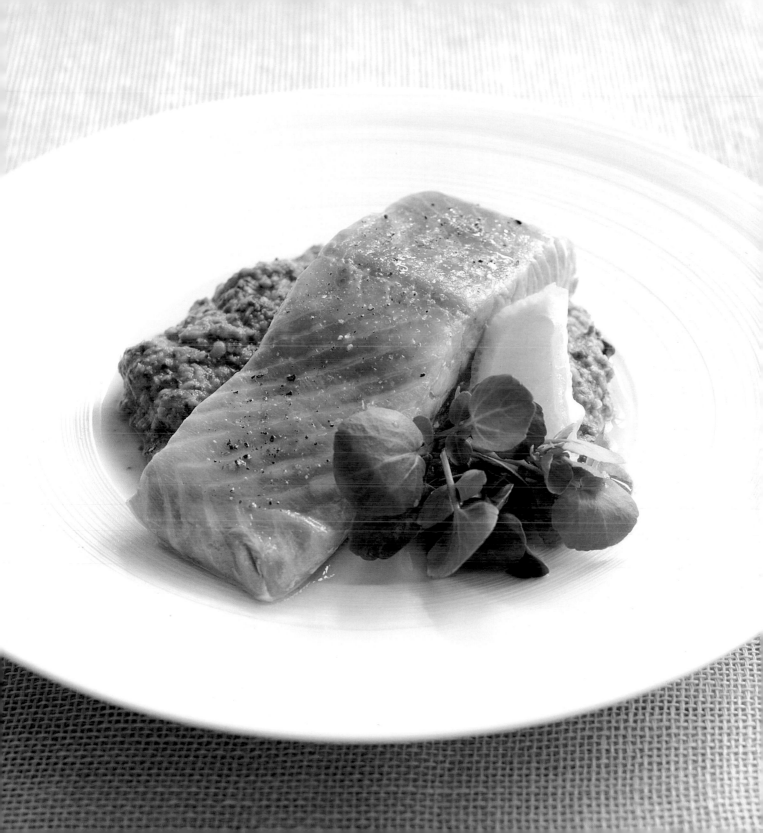

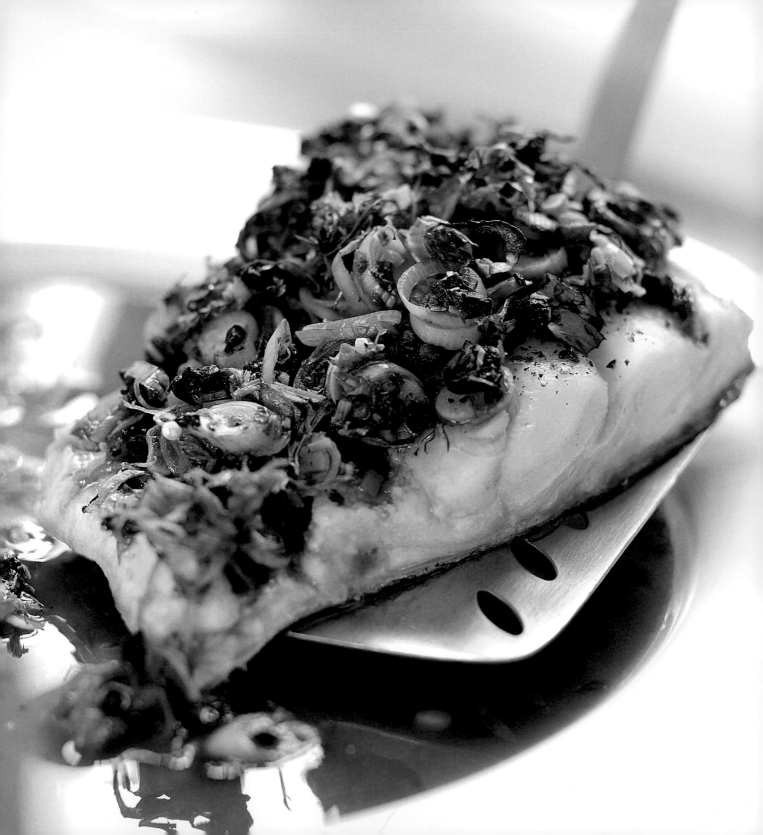

baked cod with olives and spring onions

A different way of cooking white fish. Cod is a great fish because it absorbs flavours so easily. This is a flavoursome recipe, reminiscent again of the Mediterranean. Serve with your choice of potato and a herb leaf salad.

1 teaspoon olive oil
2 x 175g cod fillets
16 black olives, pitted and finely chopped
2 tablespoons chopped parsley
1 tablespoon chopped dill
1 bunch spring onions, finely chopped
2 chillies, finely diced
Juice and zest of 1 lime
Freshly ground black pepper
150ml tomato juice
150ml fish stock

Serves 2

Preheat the oven to 230°C/450°F/gas mark 8.

Lightly oil a roasting tray and place the cod in the bottom. In a bowl, combine the olives, herbs, spring onions, chillies and lime zest with the lime juice, then spread this mixture over the top of the cod.

Season with black pepper, then pour the tomato juice and fish stock around the fish. Place on the hob and bring to the boil over a medium heat.

Place the dish in the oven and cook for 12 minutes. Serve immediately, using the juices as a sauce.

PER SERVING:
209 KCALS, 6G FAT, 1G SATURATED FAT, 5G CARBOHYDRATE, 0.92G SODIUM

roast cod with anchovy and garlic

Another oven-cooked cod dish, but with a completely different taste. Anchovies are one of my favourite flavourings and give this recipe a completely new dimension. Serve with brown rice or new potatoes.

5 tinned anchovy fillets, drained, rinsed and roughly chopped
2 teaspoons finely chopped mint
8 garlic cloves, finely chopped
4 x 200g cod steaks
3 tablespoons seasoned plain flour
2 tablespoons rapeseed oil
4 shallots, halved
2 celery sticks, finely sliced
1 carrot, finely sliced
2 tablespoons dry vermouth
400g tinned chopped tomatoes
450ml fish stock
3 tablespoons chopped parsley
Freshly ground black pepper

Serves 4

Preheat the oven to 200°C/400°F/gas mark 6.

Soak the anchovies in cold water for 30 minutes. Drain, then, in a food processor, blend the anchovies, with the mint and half the garlic to a smooth paste.

Make four 2.5cm incisions in each of the cod steaks and push the paste into the slits. Dust the cod all over with seasoned flour.

Heat the oil in a flameproof casserole dish. Brown the cod steaks all over, then remove and set aside.

Add the shallots, celery, carrot and remaining garlic to the same casserole dish, and cook until the vegetables start to soften. Return the cod to the pan and add the vermouth, tomatoes and fish stock and bring to the boil. Remove and place in the oven. Bake for 15 minutes, then fold in the parsley. Season with black pepper to taste and serve.

PER SERVING:
308 KCALS, 8G FAT, 1G SATURATED FAT, 16G CARBOHYDRATE, 0.51G SODIUM

teriyaki tuna with roast garlic noodles

Tuna lends itself to punchy flavours and this Japanese-style dish provides plenty of them. Teriyaki is a sweet-tasting sauce used to grill chicken, beef and fish.

3 tablespoons reduced-salt light soy sauce
3 tablespoons mirin or dry sherry
1 tablespoons soft brown sugar
1 tablespoon grated fresh root ginger
1 bulb garlic plus 2 garlic cloves

4 tuna steaks, about 2.5cm thick
2 tablespoons olive oil
4 spring onions, finely chopped
1 teaspoon chopped thyme
275g dried egg noodles
75g baby spinach leaves
Freshly ground black pepper

Serves 4

Preheat the oven to 190°C/375°F/gas mark 5.

In a shallow dish, combine the soy sauce, mirin or dry sherry, sugar and ginger. Finely chop the 2 garlic cloves and add to the dish. Add the tuna and cover. Refrigerate for 2 hours, turning from time to time.

Cut 5mm from the top of the garlic bulb, revealing the cut edges of the garlic cloves. Drizzle with 1 teaspoon of the olive oil, wrap in foil and roast in the oven for about 30 minutes, or until the garlic is soft, then allow to cool slightly.

Squeeze the softened garlic from each clove into a frying pan, add the remaining oil, spring onions and thyme and cook over a moderate heat until the onions are softened but not coloured.

Cook the noodles in boiling water, according to the packet instructions. Drain and tip into the garlic and onion mixture, toss to combine and fold in the spinach leaves. Toss until the spinach has wilted, and season with black pepper to taste.

Preheat the grill. Cook the tuna for 2 minutes on each side, depending on how rare you like your fish, basting with the marinade several times during cooking. Serve immediately on the noodles.

PER SERVING:
573 KCALS, 18G FAT, 4G SATURATED FAT, 57G CARBOHYDRATE, 0.71G SODIUM

spicy fish curry

We don't eat enough fish curries and I can never understand why. This dish has beautifully balanced flavours and, unlike most curries, is relatively low in fat. Serve with brown rice.

700g fish fillets (salmon, cod or monkfish)
Olive-oil spray (see page 17)
2 onions, thinly sliced
6 garlic cloves, finely diced
½ teaspoon ground coriander
½ teaspoon ground turmeric
1 teaspoon cayenne pepper
½ teaspoon ground ginger
3 tomatoes, seeded and chopped
225g leaf spinach, stems removed
Freshly ground black pepper
150g low-fat Greek yogurt

Serves 4

Cut the fish into 2.5cm cubes. Lightly spray a non-stick frying pan with olive oil, add the fish and fry until just cooked, this should take about 3 minutes. Remove and set aside.

Spray a little more oil on to the pan and fry the onions until they are soft but not coloured, then add the garlic and spices and cook for a further 5 minutes. Add the tomatoes and spinach and cook until the spinach has wilted. Season with black pepper, then add the yogurt. Bring to the boil and simmer for 5 minutes.

Return the fish to the sauce and heat through. Serve immediately with some brown rice.

PER SERVING:
328 KCALS, 14G FAT, 3G SATURATED FAT, 12G CARBOHYDRATE, 0.21G SODIUM

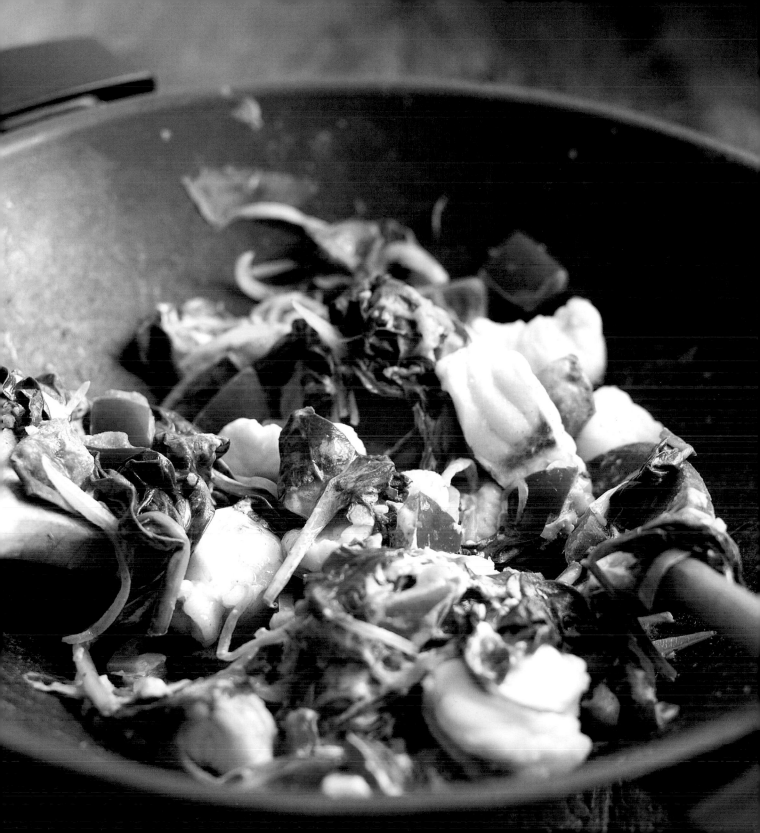

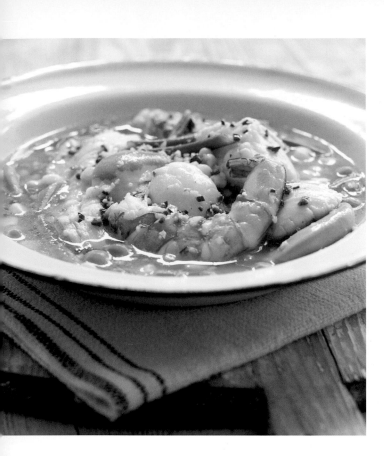

spiced fish casserole

Simple one-pot dining, inspired by the West Indies. Allspice is mainly cultivated in Jamaica and is so called because it tastes like a combination of cloves, pepper, nutmeg and cinnamon. Delicious served with some crusty bread.

½ teaspoon freshly ground black pepper
8 allspice berries, crushed
4 garlic cloves, crushed
2 hot chillies, finely chopped
Juice of 2 limes
1 tablespoon olive oil
110g monkfish
110g haddock
4 raw large prawns, shelled
4 large diver-caught scallops, shucked
600ml fish stock
75g French beans, cut into 2.5cm pieces
50g sweetcorn niblets
50g podded peas (fresh or frozen)
4 spring onions
Lime wedges, to serve

Serves 4

Combine the first 6 ingredients in a bowl to make a marinade. Place all the fish and shellfish in the marinade for 1 hour.

When ready to cook, add the fish and the shellfish with the marinade to the stock and bring to a rolling boil.

Add all the vegetables and cook for 4 minutes.

Serve the fish in bowls covered with the cooking liquid, accompanied by lime wedges.

PER SERVING:
153 KCALS, 4G FAT, 1G SATURATED FAT, 8G CARBOHYDRATE, 0.36G SODIUM

moroccan-spiced roast mackerel

Mackerel is the best-value fish on offer and has the wonderful ability to carry big flavours. It is also one of the richest sources of omega-3 fats, hence the fat content of this dish. Serve with brown rice or some new potatoes.

2 tablespoons rapeseed or olive oil
2 tablespoons chopped coriander leaves
1 teaspoon chopped mint leaves
Juice of 1 lemon
½ teaspoon chilli powder
½ teaspoon paprika
2 teaspoons ground cumin
1 teaspoon ground coriander
4 garlic cloves, crushed
½ teaspoon freshly ground black pepper
4 x 350g whole mackerel, filleted
4 tablespoons low-fat Greek yogurt

Serves 4

In a bowl, mix together the oil, chopped coriander leaves, mint, lemon juice, chilli powder, paprika, cumin, ground coriander, garlic and black pepper.

Place the mackerel fillets in the marinade and coat all over. Marinate for 30 minutes, turning from time to time.

Preheat the oven to 190°C/375°F/gas mark 5.

Place the fish and the marinade in a shallow baking dish, add 125ml water and bring to the boil on the hob. Transfer to the oven and roast for 12–15 minutes. Remove from the oven and keep warm.

Strain the cooking juices into a saucepan and fold in the yogurt. Warm through, season with black pepper and pour over the mackerel.

PER SERVING:
633 KCALS, 47G FAT, 8G SATURATED FAT, 4G CARBOHYDRATE, 0.18G SODIUM

oatmeal herrings with peppers and anchovies

Most of us only try herrings as kippers, when they have been cold-smoked, but they are best when fresh. Accompany with lower-salt dishes. Serve with a leaf salad.

4 x 350g herrings, cleaned
2 rashers lean back bacon
300ml skimmed milk
150g coarse oatmeal
Olive-oil spray (see page 17)
1 large onion, finely sliced
3 garlic cloves, finely chopped
3 tablespoons dry Martini
290g jar roasted red peppers and sun-dried tomatoes, drained and dried on kitchen paper
700g plum tomatoes, peeled and chopped
1 teaspoon chopped marjoram leaves
1 teaspoon chopped tinned capers
2 tinned anchovy fillets, drained, rinsed and chopped
16 black olives, pitted and halved

Serves 4

Preheat the oven to 200°C/400°F/gas mark 6.

Make 2 diagonal slashes in each side of each herring. Cut each rasher of bacon into 8 pieces and insert into the slashes in the herrings. Dip the herrings in the milk, then smother all over with the oatmeal.

Lightly spray a frying pan with olive oil and heat. Add the onion and garlic and cook until the onion is softened but still without colour. Add the Martini, red peppers and sun-dried tomatoes, plum tomatoes, marjoram, capers, anchovies and olives.

Simmer for 10 minutes. Tip this mixture into a baking dish, big enough to accommodate the 4 herrings.

In the same frying pan, spray with a little more olive oil and pan-fry the herrings for 1 minute on each side. Remove the herrings and place on the pepper mix and bake for 20 minutes.

PER SERVING:
754 KCALS, 44G FAT, 6G SATURATED FAT, 44G CARBOHYDRATE, 1.34G SODIUM

bouillabaisse

Entertaining in style, here are some great flavours.
This is another fantastic Mediterranean recipe that
traditionally contains several kinds of rock fish,
saffron, onions, garlic and tomatoes.

2 tablespoons olive oil
2 onions, finely chopped
4 garlic cloves, finely chopped
2 leeks, trimmed and finely chopped
1 fennel head, finely chopped, fronds reserved
400g tin chopped tomatoes
1 teaspoon fennel seeds
1 tablespoon tomato purée
1 small bunch flat-leaf parsley, separated into leaves and stalks
2 sprigs of thyme
2 bay leaves
450g fish bones (optional)
2 strips pared orange zest
600ml fish stock
500ml still mineral water
½ teaspoon saffron strands, soaked in a little warm water
4 medium floury potatoes, peeled and halved
1 tablespoon Pernod
Freshly ground black pepper
1 red mullet, scaled and filleted, each fillet halved, head and
    bones reserved
2 x 125g sea bass fillets, halved
225g monkfish fillet, cut into 4cm chunks
450g mussels, cleaned (about 20 in total)
6 raw large tiger prawns, shelled and deveined, shells reserved

Serves 4

Heat the olive oil in a large pan. Add the onions, garlic,
leeks and fennel and cook gently for 10 minutes or until the
vegetables are soft, but not coloured, stirring occasionally. Stir
in the tomatoes, fennel seeds, tomato purée, parsley stalks,
thyme and bay leaves, then add the reserved bones, if using,
and the fish trimmings and prawn shells, stirring to coat. Cook
for a minute or so, stirring until everything is well combined,
then add the orange zest and pour in the fish stock, mineral
water and saffron mixture. Bring to the boil, then reduce the
heat and simmer gently, uncovered, for 30 minutes, skimming
the surface occasionally to remove any froth. Strain and return
to the saucepan, discarding the bones and shells.

Add the potatoes to the fish broth and cook for 15 minutes.
Add the Pernod and season to taste with black pepper. Return
to a simmer, then add the red mullet and the sea bass fillets
with the monkfish and mussels. Bring back up to a simmer
and add in the prawns. Cover and cook for another 2 minutes
or until the mussels have opened and the prawns have turned
pink. Using a slotted spoon, transfer the fish and shellfish to a
warm serving platter and pour over the broth. Roughly chop
the parsley leaves and scatter on top to serve.

PER SERVING:
447 KCALS, 12G FAT, 2G SATURATED FAT, 35G CARBOHYDRATE, 0.58G SODIUM

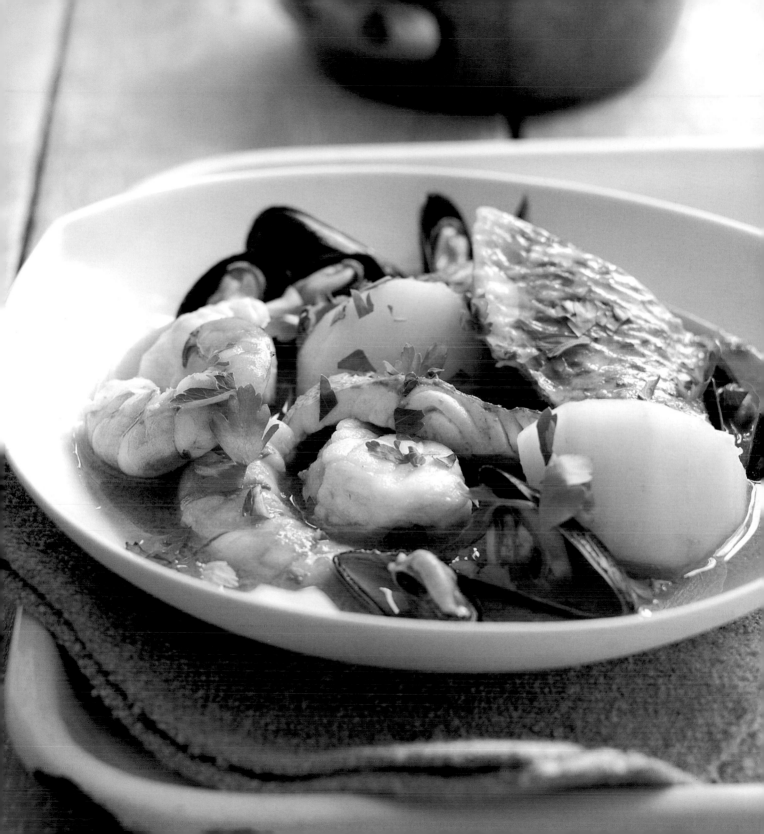

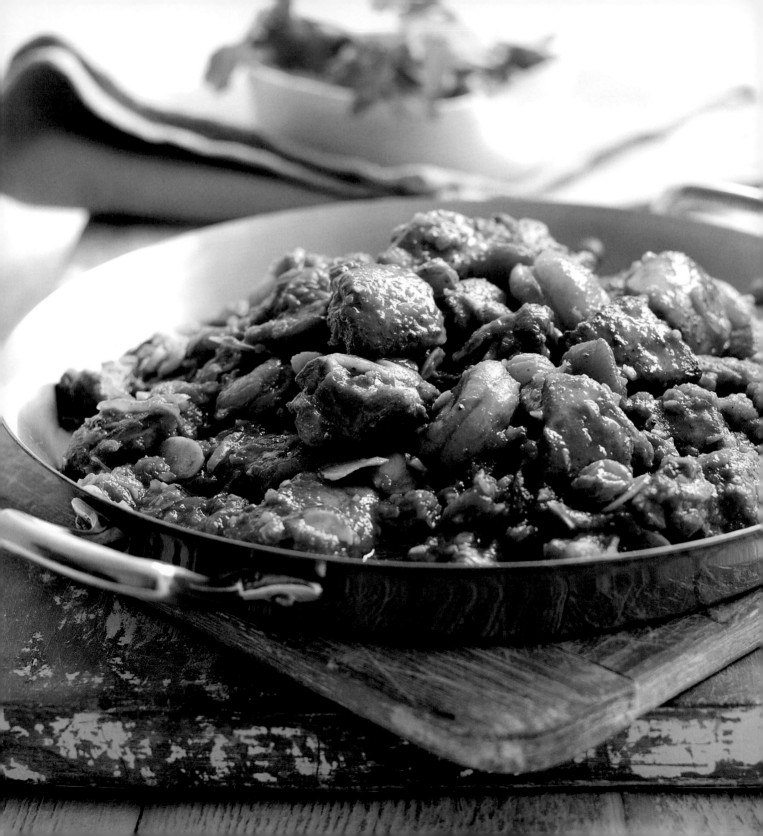

chicken tagine

Most people associate spicy with hot, but not so in this full-flavoured dish from Morocco. Made with either chicken or lamb, this stew is traditionally cooked over an open fire. Serve with Jewelled Couscous (see page 61).

½ tablespoon ground ginger
1 teaspoon freshly ground
  black pepper
½ teaspoon ground cinnamon
½ teaspoons ground turmeric
2 teaspoons paprika
½ teaspoon cayenne pepper
8 boneless, skinless chicken thighs,
  cut into 2.5cm pieces
1 tablespoon olive oil
6 garlic cloves, crushed to a paste
2 onions, grated

50g dried apricots, soaked
  in a little water
25g flaked almonds
25g sultanas or raisins
1 teaspoon runny honey
½ teaspoon saffron strands,
  soaked in a little cold water
300ml tomato juice
300ml chicken stock
400g tinned chopped
  tomatoes
2 tablespoons chopped
  coriander leaves

Serves 4

Mix all the spices together. Coat the chicken with half the spice mixture and leave overnight preferably, or for at least 2 hours.

In a heavy saucepan, heat the oil and brown the chicken over a high heat. Remove from the pan and set aside. Add the remaining spice mixture, the crushed garlic and grated onions to the pan. Allow the onions to soften without browning.

Add the apricots and their soaking water, the almonds, raisins or sultanas, honey, saffron and its liquid, tomato juice, chicken stock and tomatoes. Bring to the boil, reduce the heat to medium heat and cook until the sauce has thickened considerably, this should take about 20 minutes. Add the chicken and cook for a further 20 minutes.

Fold in the chopped coriander and serve immediately.

PER SERVING:
356 KCALS, 9G FAT, 1G SATURATED FAT, 26G CARBOHYDRATE, 0.42G SODIUM

chicken kebab tonnato

This is a fantastic grilled variation of a classic Italian veal dish, *Vitello tonnato,* which is also made with tuna and anchovies. Great for summer lunches. You could serve it with some pitta or crusty bread.

½ onion, finely diced
½ carrot, finely diced
½ celery stick, finely diced
2 garlic cloves, finely diced
½ teaspoon soft thyme leaves
1 bay leaf
2 tablespoons olive oil
110g tinned tuna in brine, drained
4 tinned anchovy fillets
150ml dry white wine
150ml chicken stock
300ml low-fat yogurt
Pinch of salt
Freshly ground black pepper
2 x 175g skinless chicken breast, cut into 1.5cm dice
Olive-oil spray (see page 17)

Serves 2

Cook the onion, carrot, celery, garlic, thyme and bay leaf in the oil until the onion is soft but not brown. Add the tuna, anchovies, white wine and stock and simmer for 20 minutes or until 100ml liquid remains. Remove the bay leaf and blend the mixture in a food processor until smooth.

Allow to cool, then fold in the yogurt. Season with black pepper to taste.

Thread the chicken on to 4 satay or cocktail sticks, spray lightly with oil and grill for 3 minutes on each side. Season with a little salt and black pepper. Serve the hot kebabs with the cold tuna sauce.

PER SERVING:
501 KCALS, 16G FAT, 3G SATURATED FAT, 15G CARBOHYDRATE, 0.94G SODIUM

the really useful chicken recipe

This is exactly what it says it is: a really healthy way of cooking chicken that is delicious on its own or used in salads (see Asian chicken salad, page 73), sandwiches or stew.

1.5kg free-range chicken, skin removed
4 spring onions, sliced
3 x 5mm discs fresh root ginger
6 garlic cloves, peeled
1 chilli
10 black peppercorns

Serves 4

Place the chicken in a saucepan with a tightly fitting lid, cover with water and add the remaining ingredients.

Bring to the boil and simmer for 35 minutes, turning the chicken once during the cooking process. Cover with a lid and turn off the heat. Allow the chicken to relax in the liquid for 1 hour.

Remove the chicken. Allow to cool completely, then cut up and use as required.

PER SERVING:
212 KCALS, 8G FAT, 3G SATURATED FAT, 0G CARBOHYDRATE, 0.09G SODIUM

grilled chicken with coriander chutney

A very simple meal, quick to make and with lots of taste. Whenever possible, buy organic chicken as the flavour is noticeably better.

Olive-oil spray (see page 17)
2 x 175g skinless chicken breasts
175g basmati rice, cooked

For the chutney
25g mint leaves
25g coriander leaves
1 small onion, roughly chopped
1.5cm fresh root ginger, peeled and grated
1 chilli, roughly chopped
½ teaspoon cumin seeds
1 garlic clove
2 teaspoons lemon juice
1 tablespoon desiccated coconut, moistened in a little water

Serves 2

To make the chutney, blend the ingredients in a food processor until smooth.

Lightly spray the chicken breasts with oil and cook under a hot grill for 8 minutes on each side. Serve the chicken with the chutney, basmati rice and a leaf salad.

PER SERVING:
546 KCALS, 7G FAT, 4G SATURATED FAT, 75G CARBOHYDRATE, 0.12G SODIUM

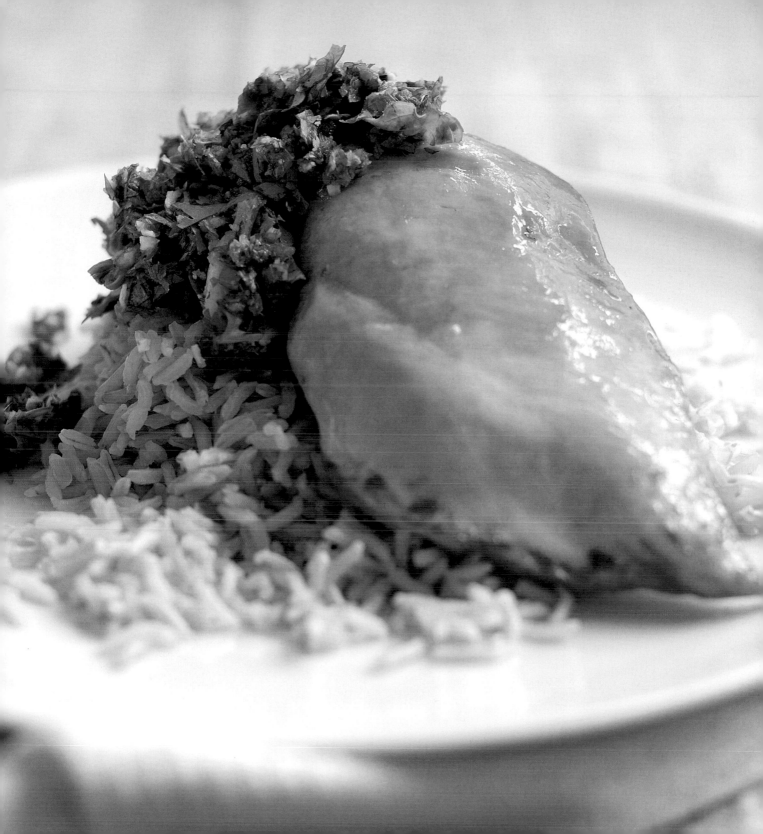

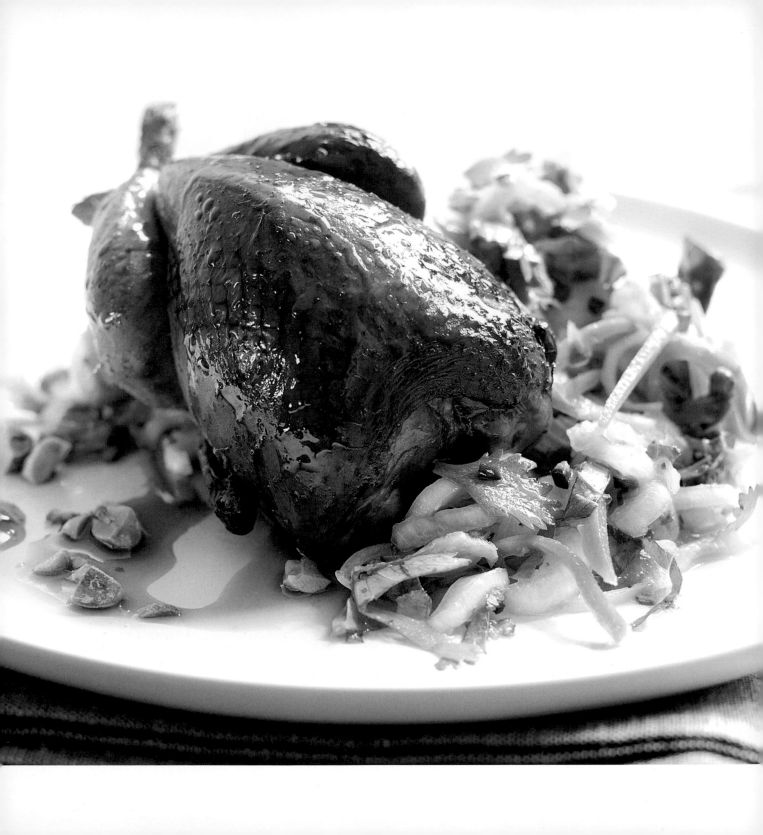

tea-smoked quail

Home smoking at its easiest: the tea, sugar and rice make a simple smoking mixture, while the Asian marinade gives fantastic flavour. It also contains much less salt than bought smoked food. Serve with roasted vegetables and brown rice for a main dish.

1 tablespoon sesame oil
2 tablespoons runny honey
1 tablespoon reduced-salt soy sauce
4 quail
2 tablespoons jasmine tea leaves
2 tablespoons demerara sugar
2 tablespoons rice

Serves 2 (4 as a starter)

Combine the sesame oil, honey and soy sauce in a bowl, rub over the quail and marinate for 1 hour.

Make a smoking mixture by combining the tea leaves, sugar and rice. Cut a circle of foil that will fit the bottom of a wok, and scrunch the sides until you have made a container about 12cm in diameter. Place it in the bottom of the wok and put the smoking mixture in the bottom.

Place the wok over the highest heat and, once the mixture starts to smoke, place the quail on a circular metal rack that fits half-way up the wok. Cover with a tight-fitting lid and smoke for 5 minutes.

Remove the wok from the heat and allow the quail to continue to smoke without lifting the lid for 1–2 minutes.

Serve with Asian slaw (see page 70).

PER SERVING:
461 KCALS, 29G FAT, 7G SATURATED FAT, 4G CARBOHYDRATE, 0.22G SODIUM

asian pork in lettuce leaves

A lovely way of serving and eating pork. The light Oriental flavours and the fresh crunch of the lettuce leaves make this a delicious meal, hot or cold.

2 garlic cloves, finely chopped
½ heaped teaspoon freshly ground black pepper
Juice and zest of 1 lime
2 tablespoons chopped coriander leaves
1 tablespoon groundnut or sunflower oil
225g lean minced pork
1 tablespoon chopped unsalted peanuts
2 tablespoons chopped tinned bamboo shoots
1 tablespoon nam pla (Thai fish sauce) or reduced-salt light soy sauce
1 teaspoon runny honey
1 bird's eye chilli, finely chopped
2 shallots, thinly sliced
2 large oranges, segmented
2 tablespoons chopped mint
2 little gem lettuces, separated into leaves

Serves 2

Heat a large frying pan or wok. Mix together the garlic, pepper, lime juice and zest and half of the coriander in a bowl. Add the oil to the pan, tip in the garlic mixture and stir-fry for 30 seconds. Add the pork and stir-fry for 8–10 minutes until well browned, breaking up the mince with a wooden spoon as it cooks.

Add the peanuts, bamboo shoots, fish sauce or soy sauce, honey and chilli to the pork mixture and cook for another 5 minutes or until the liquid has almost completely evaporated, stirring occasionally. Season to taste.

Place the shallots in a bowl with the orange segments and a heaped teaspoon each of the mint and remaining coriander. Mix until well combined and pile into the middle of a large plate or platter. Stir in the remaining mint and coriander into the pork mixture and use to fill the lettuce leaves, arranging them around the orange salad.

Place a little of the orange salad on top of each pork parcel and eat immediately.

PER SERVING:
336 KCALS, 14G FAT, 3G SATURATED FAT, 23G CARBOHYDRATE, 0.62G SODIUM

rice bake with pancetta, greens and pecans

A really substantial meal, especially as most of the fat is unsaturated. This rice bake is great served with a leaf salad.

1.5 litres chicken stock
1 bay leaf
1 sprig thyme
225g brown rice
25g margarine
115g pancetta or lean smoked streaky bacon, roughly chopped
2 onions, finely chopped
3 celery sticks, finely chopped
½ Savoy cabbage, chopped
3 tablespoons finely chopped marjoram
½ sachet sage and onion stuffing
110g chopped pecans
Freshly ground black pepper
2 eggs, beaten
Olive-oil spray (see page 17)

Serves 6

Bring 850ml of the stock, the bay leaf and thyme to the boil. Add the rice, reduce the heat, cover and cook for 30 minutes. Transfer the rice to a large bowl, discarding the bay leaf and thyme.

Meanwhile, melt the margarine in a large saucepan, add the pancetta or bacon, onions and celery. Cook over a medium heat for 8 minutes until the onions are soft but not brown. Add the cabbage and marjoram and cook for 5 minutes, stirring regularly. Add this mixture to the rice, fold in the stuffing, pecans, plenty of black pepper and the beaten eggs.

Lightly oil a large baking dish. Fold the remaining chicken stock into the stuffing and place in the baking dish. Cover with oiled foil and bake in a hot oven for 30 minutes.

PER SERVING:
425 KCALS, 25G FAT, 4G SATURATED FAT, 39G CARBOHYDRATE, 0.69G SODIUM

ham bollito with salsa verde

Bollito misto usually contains several meats (it means 'boiled mixed' in Italian), but this ham version is just as delicious. It is traditionally served with salsa verde.

4 small carrots, peeled and left whole
4 small onions, peeled, with root intact
1.5kg ham joint, soaked overnight in water and drained
2 celery hearts, quartered through the root end
12 black peppercorns
3 fresh bay leaves
Pared rind of 1 orange, studded with 4 whole cloves
12 parsley stalks
12 new salad potatoes (such as Charlotte) unpeeled
120g podded broad beans (fresh or frozen)
12 baby leeks, trimmed
Salsa Verde (see page 62), to serve

Serves 8

Put the carrots and onions into a pan large enough to hug the ham joint and place the ham joint on top. Add the celery, peppercorns, bay leaves and studded orange rind, then add enough water so that the liquid covers the ham completely.

Add the parsley stalks to the pan and bring to the boil. Reduce the heat and simmer for 1 hour, skimming off any scum that rises to the top and topping up with boiling water as required to keep the ham completely covered. Cook the ham following the instructions on the wrapping – about 20 minutes per 450g.

Add the new potatoes 20 minutes before the end of the cooking time. Add the broad beans and leeks 10 minutes before the end. Discard the orange and parsley stalks.

Remove the ham from the pan and place on a carving board. Snip away the string and cut away any excess fat, then carve into thick slices. Arrange the ham slices on serving plates and spoon around a selection of the vegetables and a little broth. Serve with Salsa Verde and Dijon mustard.

PER SERVING:
267 KCALS, 7G FAT, 2G SATURATED FAT, 12G CARBOHYDRATE, 1.39G SODIUM

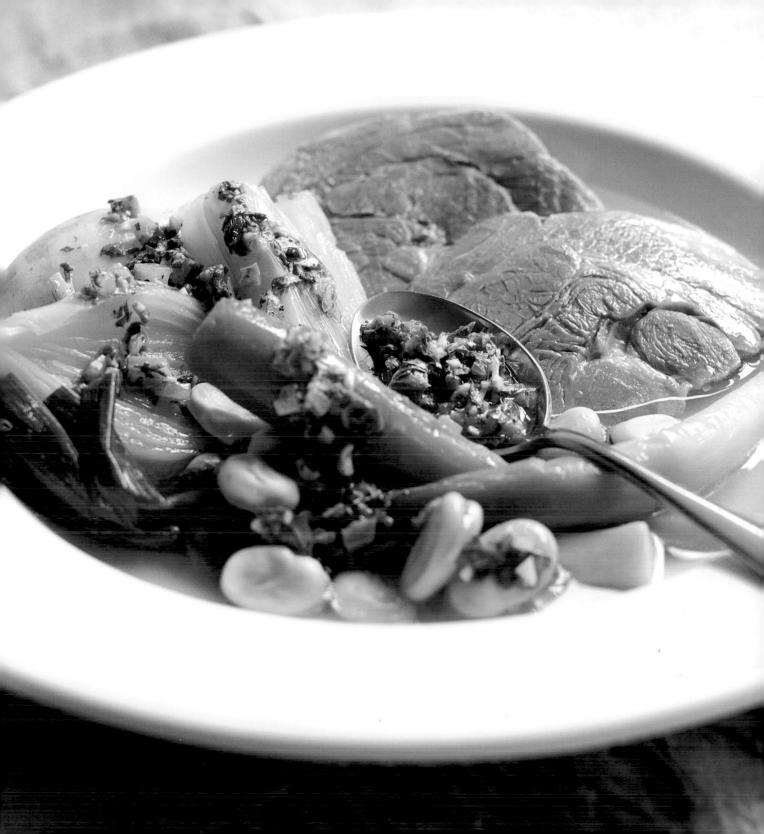

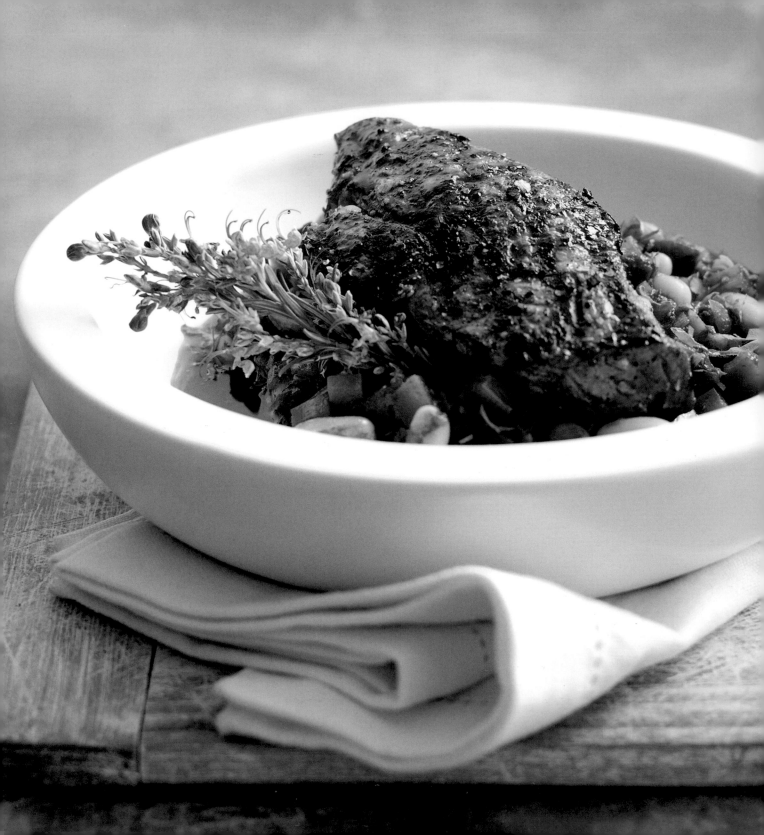

tuscan-style lamb

Here are more wonderful flavours from Italy. This is a really nutritious dish filled with the Mediterranean staples – tomatoes, beans, fish, olive oil and garlic.

2 lamb chumps, fat and skin removed
9 small sprigs of rosemary
4 garlic cloves, finely chopped
Freshly ground black pepper
Olive-oil spray (see page 17)
1 onion, finely chopped
2 carrots, diced
2 celery sticks, diced

1 heaped teaspoon thyme leaves
4 tinned anchovy fillets, rinsed, drained and finely chopped
125ml red wine
300ml lamb or chicken stock
400g chopped tomatoes
1 tablespoon tomato purée
400g tinned cannellini beans, drained and rinsed
2 tablespoons chopped parsley

Serves 2

Toss the lamb chumps with the rosemary and half the garlic and season with black pepper. Place in a non-metallic dish. Cover with clingfilm and leave for 1 hour at room temperature or up to 24 hours in a fridge.

Heat a sauté pan, lightly spray with olive oil and fry the onion, carrots, celery and thyme over a high heat for about 10 minutes, stirring regularly until softened and lightly browned, then stir in the remaining garlic and the anchovies.

Pour in the red wine, scraping the bottom of the pan with a wooden spoon to release any sediment, then add the stock, tomatoes and tomato purée. Season with black pepper, bring to the boil, then reduce the heat and simmer for another 15–20 minutes until well reduced and thickened, stirring occasionally. Heat a griddle pan, barbecue or grill and cook the chumps for 5 minutes on each side until lightly charred and medium-rare. Season with black pepper.

Add the beans and most of the parsley to the tomato mixture and stir to combine. Season with black pepper and cook for 5 minutes or until heated through. Spoon into wide-rimmed bowls, garnish with the rest of the parsley and arrange the lamb chumps on top to serve.

PER SERVING:
606 KCALS, 22G FAT, 7G SATURATED FAT, 44G CARBOHYDRATE, 0.9G SODIUM

lamb kofta with spiced yogurt

The Middle East uses great spices to flavour its food and lamb absorbs them so well. The spicy meatballs and minty yogurt are an irresistible combination. Serve with wholemeal pitta bread.

75g bulghur cracked wheat
2 tablespoons olive oil
1 chilli, finely chopped
1 medium onion, finely chopped
½ teaspoon ground coriander
½ teaspoon ground cumin
500g leg of lamb, lean, all visible fat removed, diced
1 egg
40g pine kernels, finely chopped

2 tablespoons chopped mint
2 tablespoons chopped parsley

For the spiced yogurt
2 chillies, seeded and finely chopped
1 tablespoon chopped mint
1 tablespoon snipped chives
1 tablespoon coriander leaves, finely chopped
1 tablespoon finely chopped parsley
1 garlic clove, crushed to a paste
½ teaspoon ground cumin
250g low-fat Greek yogurt

Makes 40

Soak the bulghur in cold water for 30 minutes, drain and squeeze dry.

Heat half the olive oil in a frying pan, then add the chilli, onion, ground coriander and cumin and cook over a low heat for 15 minutes. Drain, retaining the oil, and allow to cool.

Beat the egg. Place the lamb in a food processor with the egg and the onion mix and blend to a smooth paste. Remove and place in a bowl with the cracked wheat, pine kernels and herbs. Wet your hands and shape 1 teaspoon of the mixture into a small ball. Repeat to make 40 balls in total.

To make the spiced yogurt, combine all the ingredients together and leave for an hour to allow the flavours to develop.

Add the remaining oil to the reserved oil in a frying pan. Over a medium heat, fry the kofta in batches, turning regularly until brown and cooked through, this should take about 10 minutes. Keep warm in the oven. Repeat until all the kofta are cooked. Drain the kofta on absorbent kitchen paper and serve with the spiced yogurt dip.

PER SERVING (4 KOFTA):
188 KCALS, 12G FAT, 4G SATURATED FAT, 8G CARBOHYDRATE, 0.08G SODIUM

shepherd's pie with a difference

Here, the cauliflower topping makes an unusual and healthier change from the traditional mashed potato. A classic English recipe.

Olive-oil spray (see page 17)
1 large onion, finely chopped
450g lean minced lamb
1 tablespoon plain flour
2 bay leaves
1 teaspoon chopped thyme
1 teaspoon anchovy essence
200g tinned chopped tomatoes
250ml lamb, chicken or beef stock
2 teaspoons Worcestershire sauce
Freshly ground black pepper
For the topping
1 medium cauliflower, broken into florets
2 tablespoons low-fat Greek yogurt
1 egg yolk
2 tablespoons soft wholegrain breadcrumbs

Serves 4

Heat a frying pan. Spray lightly with olive oil, then tip in the onion and cook for 5 minutes until softened but not browned, stirring occasionally.

Meanwhile, heat a large, heavy-based pan and spray lightly with olive oil. Tip in half the minced lamb and cook over a fairly high heat until evenly browned, breaking up any lumps with the back of a wooden spoon and straining off any melted fat. Transfer to a plate. Cook the rest of the lamb, then return all of the lamb to the pan, adding the cooked onions and stirring to combine.

Sprinkle over the flour and then add the bay leaves, thyme and anchovy essence, stirring to combine. Add the chopped tomatoes, stock, Worcestershire sauce and a good pinch of pepper. Bring to the boil, then reduce the heat, cover and simmer for 45 minutes–1 hour until the lamb is completely tender and softened. Season with black pepper. Allow to cool, then refrigerate. Remove any solidified fat from the top. Preheat the oven to 180°C/350°F/gas mark 4.

Meanwhile, to make the topping, place the cauliflower in a pan of boiling water, cover and simmer for 15–20 minutes or until tender. Drain and return to the pan for a couple of minutes to dry out, shaking the pan occasionally to prevent the cauliflower sticking to the bottom. Place the cauliflower in a food processor and blend until smooth. Place in a large bowl and beat in the yogurt and egg yolk. Season with black pepper to taste.

Spoon the lamb mixture into a 1.8 litre pie dish, discarding the bay leaves. Cover with the mashed cauliflower, then smooth over and mark with a spatula. Top with the breadcrumbs and spray with a little oil. Bake for 25–30 minutes or until bubbling and golden brown. Serve at once straight from the dish with a bowl of peas, if liked.

PER SERVING:
303 KCALS, 13G FAT, 5G SATURATED FAT, 16G CARBOHYDRATE, 0.34G SODIUM

lancashire hotpot with sweet potatoes

Another traditional dish with a twist. Sweet potatoes contain more beta-carotene than ordinary potatoes. Use water instead of stock if you want to reduce the fat and sodium.

4 lamb's kidneys, skinned
8 x 110g lamb chump chops, excess fat removed
1 heaped tablespoon plain flour
Freshly ground black pepper
½ tablespoon sunflower oil
600ml fresh lamb stock
Olive-oil spray (see page 17)
750g sweet potatoes, peeled
1 large floury potato, peeled
4 sprigs of thyme
2 onions, thinly sliced
2 fresh bay leaves

Serves 4

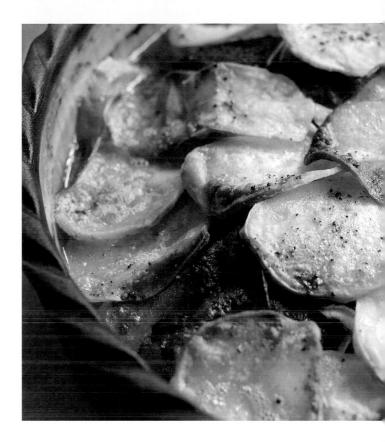

Preheat the oven to 180°C/350°F/gas mark 4.

Place the kidneys on a chopping board and cut each one in half, then, using a small pair of scissors, remove the central core and membrane. Place in a bowl with the lamb chops, add the flour and season generously with black pepper. Toss to coat, shaking off any excess.

Heat a large non-stick frying pan. Add the oil and brown the chops for 2–3 minutes on each side – you may have to do this in batches depending on the size of the pan. Transfer to a plate and set aside. Add the kidneys to the frying pan and fry for 1–2 minutes on each side, then add to the plate with the chops. Tip away any excess fat from the pan, then add a little of the stock to deglaze, scraping the bottom with a wooden spoon to remove any sediment.

Spray a heavy-based 4.5 litre casserole dish with a little oil. Cut the sweet potatoes into 1cm slices. Thinly slice the floury potato and set aside for the top of the hotpot.

Line the bottom of the dish with half of the sweet potato slices. Place four of the chops on top, then add 2 thyme sprigs and half of the onions. Season with black pepper to taste and pop the kidneys around the sides of the casserole dish. Repeat the layers with the remaining ingredients and then pour over the stock used to deglaze the pan together with the remaining stock.

Finally, arrange an overlapping layer of the floury potato on top. Spray a little olive oil over the potato, cover and bake in the oven for 2½ hours until the lamb is completely tender, removing the lid for the final 30 minutes to allow the potatoes to go golden brown.

Serve the Lancashire hotpot straight from the casserole dish with bowls of steamed broccoli and carrots.

PER SERVING:
569 KCALS, 18G FAT, 8G SATURATED FAT, 53G CARBOHYDRATE, 0.5G SODIUM

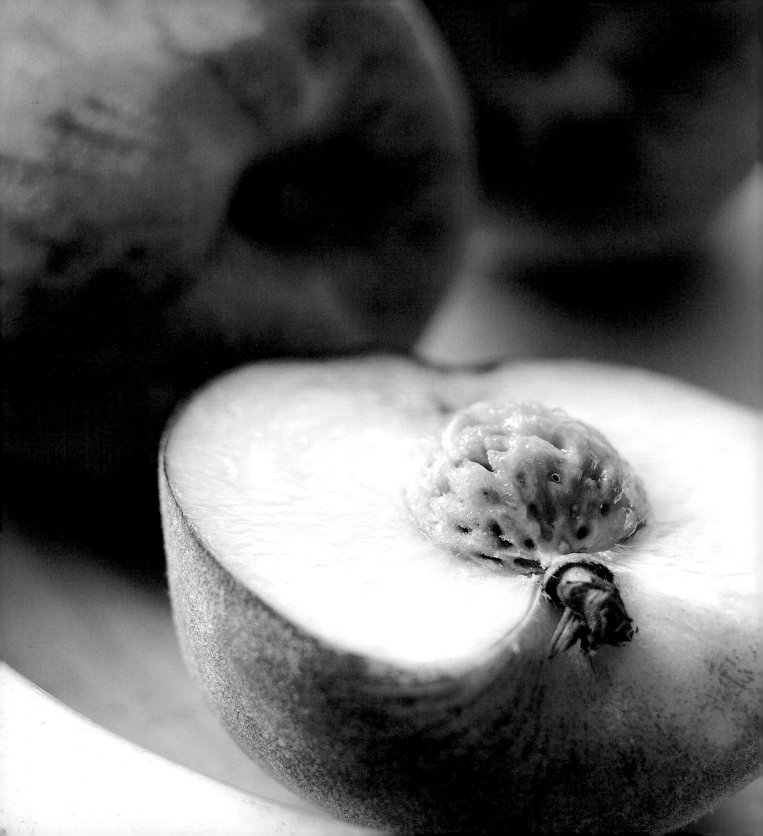

5

desserts

peach and blueberry gratin

So simple, so delicious, this gratin should evoke gasps of delight and anticipation from your guests. This is an elegant dessert that won't cause you too much stress to make.

4 tinned peach halves in natural juice
75g blueberries
50g mascarpone cheese
175g low-fat Greek yogurt
1 tablespoon caster sugar
½ teaspoon ground cinnamon

Serves 4

Place the peach halves in the bottom of 4 ramekin dishes and top with the blueberries.

Beat together the mascarpone and yogurt with a wooden spoon, then pour it over the fruit. Combine the sugar and cinnamon, then sprinkle over the yogurt mix.

Preheat the grill to its highest setting. Place the ramekins under the grill for 5–6 minutes until the sugar is golden. Alternatively, glaze using a cook's blow torch, chef-style. Allow to cool for a couple of minutes and serve.

PER SERVING:
133 KCALS, 8G FAT, 5G SATURATED FAT, 12G CARBOHYDRATE, 0.05G SODIUM

raspberry-ripple zabaglione

A wonderfully light and moussy custard, adorned with fresh raspberries. The slightly sharp taste of the fruit adds a little zing to this dessert.

225g raspberries
Juice of ½ lemon
2 teaspoons icing sugar
4 egg yolks
1 tablespoon caster sugar
2 tablespoons medium-dry sherry
2 tablespoons dry white wine
4 tablespoons low-fat Greek yogurt

Serves 4

Reserve 12 raspberries for decoration and place the rest in a food processor with a good squeeze of lemon juice. Blitz to a purée, then push through a sieve to remove the seeds. Add icing sugar to taste, leaving the fruit slightly on the tart side, then set aside.

Place the egg yolks and caster sugar in a large, heatproof bowl. Beat in the sherry and wine, using a balloon whisk. Place over a pan of simmering water and heat gently, whisking continuously until the mixture is very light but holds its shape. When it is the consistency of semi-melted ice cream, take it off the heat and continue to whisk over a bowl of iced water until cool – this prevents it from splitting.

Fold the yogurt into the mixture. Drizzle in the raspberry purée and gently swirl to create a ripple effect. Spoon into stemmed serving glasses, decorate with the reserved raspberries and serve with wafer-thin biscuits, if you like.

PER SERVING:
126 KCALS, 6G FAT, 2G SATURATED FAT, 10G CARBOHYDRATE, 0.02G SODIUM

mango fool with mango sauce

Mango and lime is a truly wonderful marriage of flavours. This refreshing dessert is especially welcome after a heavy meal.

2 egg yolks
25g caster sugar
2 tablespoons Kirsch (optional)
Juice of 2 limes
175ml low-fat Greek yogurt
2 mangoes, peeled, stoned and puréed

Serves 4

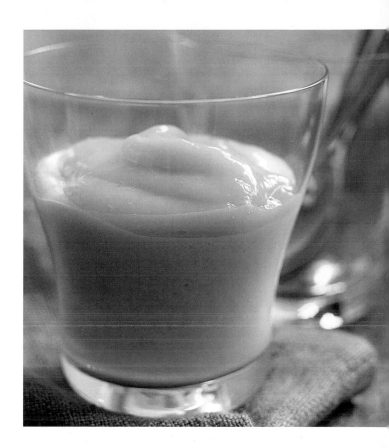

Place a bowl over a saucepan of simmering water, add the egg yolks and sugar and beat until the mixture has thickened and trebled in volume, this should take about 10 minutes. Remove the bowl and sit it over ice. Whisk until cold, then place in the refrigerator.

When cool, add half the Kirsch (if using) and half the lime juice. In a separate bowl, whip the yogurt lightly and fold into two-thirds of the mango purée. Fold this into the egg mixture. Pour into glasses or bowls and refrigerate.

Whisk the remaining Kirsch (if using), lime juice and mango purée together and pour over the mango fool to serve.

PER SERVING:
177 KCALS, 5G FAT, 2G SATURATED FAT, 29G CARBOHYDRATE, 0.04G SODIUM

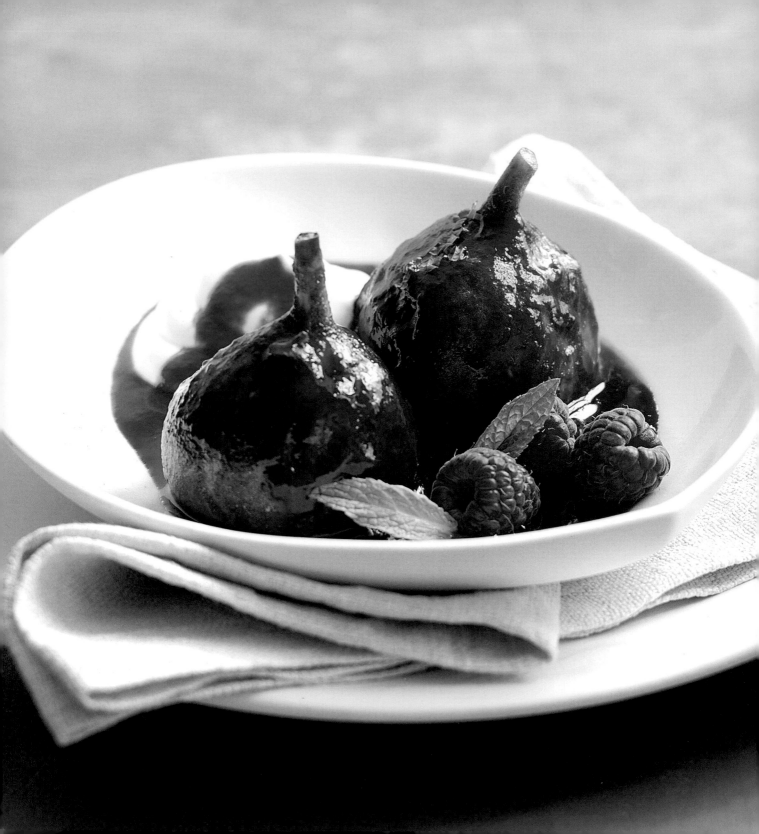

poached figs with raspberries in red wine

Figs have found more favour in savoury food of late, but this dish returns them to their rightful puddingy place.

450g ripe raspberries or blackberries
Juice of 2 lemons
Juice of 1 orange
50g caster sugar
1 glass Zinfandel red wine
8 firm fresh figs
3 tablespoons crème de mure (blackberry liqueur) or crème de cassis (blackcurrant liqueur) – optional
1 tablespoon freshly chopped mint
Low-fat fromage frais, to serve

Serves 4

Place the berries in a food processor with the lemon and orange juice and process until smooth. Strain the purée through a fine sieve into a non-reactive (not aluminium) saucepan. Discard the pips.

Add the sugar and the red wine to the berry purée and place the pan over a medium heat. Bring to the boil and simmer gently, skimming off any scum that might rise to the surface. When the sugar has dissolved, add the figs and poach for 5–6 minutes depending on their ripeness. Remove the figs to a glass bowl when cooked.

Reduce the berry cooking liquor to approximately 300ml. Allow to cool. Add the crème de mure or cassis, if using, and mint and pour over the figs. Cover and chill overnight. Serve with low-fat fromage frais.

PER SERVING:
153 KCALS, 0.6G FAT, 0G SATURATED FAT, 31G CARBOHYDRATE, 0.01G SODIUM

nutty apple tart with a twist

The combination of Granny Smith and Bramley apples, sweet and tart, works well here, while the cinnamon and cloves add a touch of the exotic to a classic dish.

4 Granny Smith apples, peeled, halved and cored
Juice of 1 lemon
2 Bramley apples, peeled, cored and diced
50g caster sugar
½ teaspoon ground cinnamon
½ teaspoon ground cloves
225g ready-made short-crust pastry
25g hazelnuts, toasted and chopped
1 egg, beaten
1 tablespoon icing sugar

Serves 6

Place the Granny Smith apples in a bowl with the lemon juice and pour in enough water to cover. Place the Bramley apples in a saucepan with 3 tablespoons water, cover and simmer for 20 minutes, stirring occasionally. Remove the lid and beat in the caster sugar, cinnamon and cloves until you have a smooth purée. Remove from the heat and leave to cool completely.

Roll the pastry on a lightly floured work surface to a 23cm square, then trim the edges. Transfer to a baking sheet lined with non-stick baking paper and chill for at least 30 minutes. Drain the Granny Smith apples and slice each half into 8 thin slices. Preheat the oven to 200°C/400°F/gas mark 6.

Remove the pastry from the fridge and spread the purée over the pastry using a spatula, leaving a 1cm border around the edges. Sprinkle on the hazelnuts, then top with the apple slices in overlapping layers. Brush the border of the pastry with the beaten egg. Bake for 15–20 minutes or until the pastry is puffed up and golden brown and the apple slices are tender and lightly golden.

Remove the tart from the oven and sprinkle over enough icing sugar to cover the apple slices. Using a cook's blow torch, caramelise the apples; alternatively place the tart under a very hot grill for a few seconds. Cut the tart into slices and serve with a little vanilla custard (see page 135), if liked.

PER SERVING:
308 KCALS, 14G FAT, 6G SATURATED FAT, 43G CARBOHYDRATE, 0.08G SODIUM

pineapple carpaccio with a fruit 'daiquiri' sauce

Thin slices of pineapple in a fruity cocktail. This dessert is as low in fat as it is high in flavour.

1 medium pineapple, peeled, cored and 'eyes' removed
2 ripe bananas, peeled
125g ripe strawberries, hulled
3 tablespoons low-fat Greek yogurt
2 tablespoons dark rum
1 tablespoon honey
4 sprigs of mint

Serves 4

Using a sharp knife, cut the pineapple into paper-thin slices and arrange them so they cover the base of four large plates.

In a liquidiser, blend together the bananas, strawberries (reserving 4 for decoration), yogurt, rum and honey until smooth.

Slice the 4 reserved strawberries. Drizzle the fruit sauce over the pineapple and decorate with the strawberries and mint sprigs.

PER SERVING:
157 KCALS, 1G FAT, 1G SATURATED FAT, 32G CARBOHYDRATE, 0.02G SODIUM

fruit salad with kiwi juices

Here's a fruit salad with a twist – the sweet, slightly spicy wine complements the fruits admirably. Something for the summer: light, fruity and very moreish.

300ml Gerwurztraminer wine
2 tablespoons runny honey
6 kiwi fruit, peeled
2 Granny Smith apples, peeled and cored
2 tablespoons lemon juice
1 mango, peeled, stoned and diced
10 large strawberries, hulled and halved
½ pineapple, peeled, cored, 'eyes' removed and cubed

Serves 4

Bring the wine and honey to the boil and then allow to cool to room temperature.

In a food processor, blend 4 of the kiwi fruit with the wine and honey mix. If you don't like the seeds of kiwi fruit, pass through a fine sieve. Cut each of the remaining kiwi into 8 wedges.

Dice the apples and toss with the lemon juice. Combine with the other fruits.

Arrange the fruit salad in the centre of your bowl, ladle the kiwi juice around them, and chill until ready to eat. Serve with the kiwi wedges.

PER SERVING:
253 KCALS, 1G FAT, 0G SATURATED FAT, 50G CARBOHYDRATE, 0.02G SODIUM

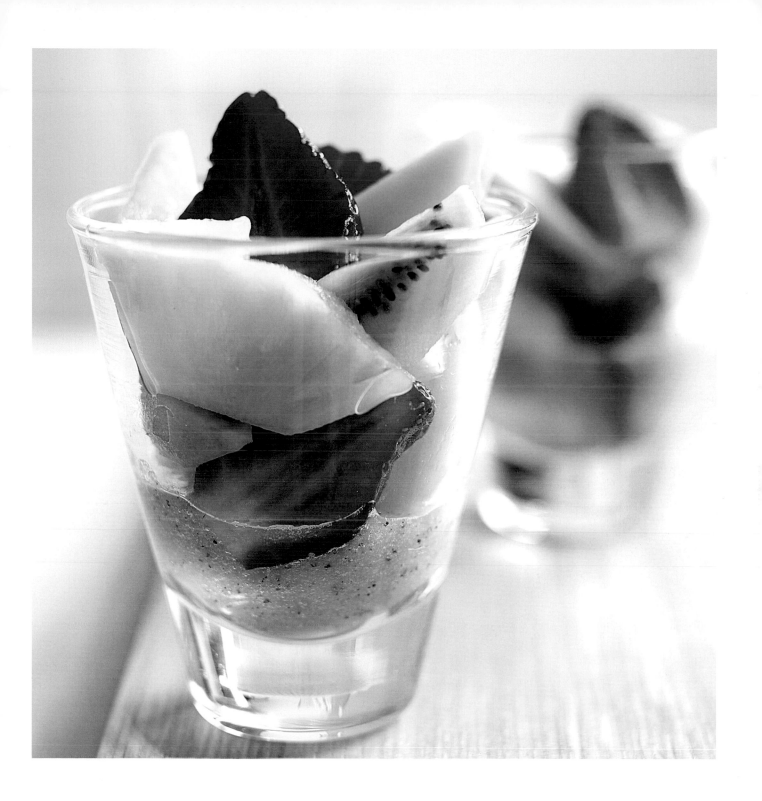

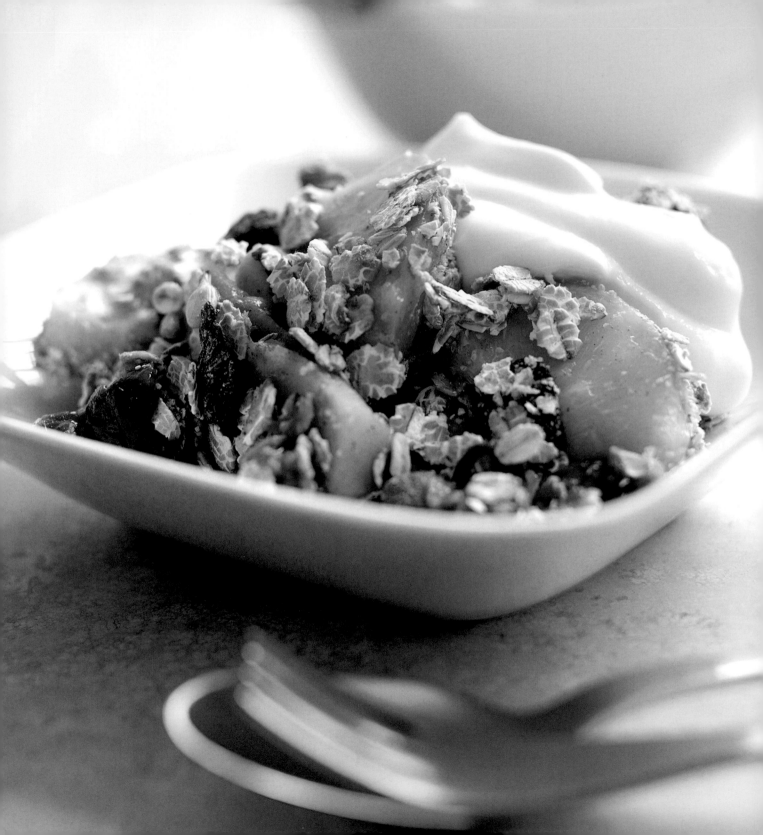

fruity apple crisp

Miss your crumble? This is the next best thing. Full of fruit and spice and all things nice, the muesli or granola makes a wonderfully crispy, yet healthy topping.

3 Granny Smith apples, peeled, cored and each cut into 8
2 peaches, peeled, stoned and each cut into 6
50g mixed dried fruits (cranberries, blueberries, cherries)
1 tablespoon soft brown muscovado sugar
½ teaspoon ground cinnamon
½ teaspoon apple pie spice
Juice and grated zest of 1 orange
2 tablespoons plain flour
175g unsweetened muesli or granola

Serves 6

Preheat the oven to 180°C/350°F/gas mark 4.

Combine all the ingredients except the muesli or granola and spoon into a baking dish. Sprinkle with the muesli or granola and bake in the oven for about 45 minutes until golden and the fruit is bubbling. Serve with Vanilla Custard (see right).

PER SERVING:
203 KCALS, 3G FAT, 0.4G SATURATED FAT, 43G CARBOHYDRATE, 0.02G SODIUM

vanilla custard

A classic custard, this is the healthy version that you will turn to again and again. The vanilla pods give it a seductive fragrance. Serve with your favourite fruity puddings.

2 tablespoons cornflour
4 teaspoons caster sugar
600ml skimmed milk
1 vanilla pod or 1 teaspoon vanilla extract
2 egg yolks

Serves 4

Mix the cornflour and sugar with a little milk to form a paste, then add the remaining milk.

Split the vanilla pod lengthways and, with the tip of a small knife, scrape the seeds into the milk, then pop the pods into the milk as well, or add the vanilla extract instead.

Cook the milk over a low heat until the mixture boils and thickens. Remove the vanilla pods, if using, and slowly whisk the milk into the egg yolks. Return to the heat and cook very slowly, stirring continuously until the custard coats the back of the spoon. Do not allow to boil. Serve hot or cold.

PER SERVING:
129 KCALS, 3G FAT, 1G SATURATED FAT, 20G CARBOHYDRATE, 0.09G SODIUM

fruity rice pudding

This pudding has nothing in common with school-dinner rice puddings. The real deal, full of flavour and fruit, and made with brown rice for extra fibre.

100g brown rice, washed
350ml skimmed milk
4 medium eggs
25g margarine, softened
75g caster sugar
75g mixed dried fruits (cranberries, cherries, blueberries, sultanas)
½ teaspoon ground cinnamon
125g raspberries

Serves 6

Bring the rice and milk to the boil in a saucepan, then reduce the heat and cook, covered, until most of the milk has evaporated into the rice, this should take about 1½ hours.

Preheat the oven to 180°C/350°F/gas mark 4.

In a bowl, beat the eggs. Fold the eggs into the rice, a little at a time, then add the margarine and the sugar.

Dust the dried fruits with cinnamon, then add them to the rice mixture.

Put a few raspberries in the bottom of 6 ramekins, then spoon the rice over the raspberries. Place the ramekins in a roasting tray and pour warm water in the tray until it reaches half-way up the sides of the ramekins. Bake in the oven for 50 minutes, and eat hot or cold.

PER SERVING:
248 KCALS, 8G FAT, 2G SATURATED FAT, 39G CARBOHYDRATE, 0.11G SODIUM

chocolate steamed pudding

Everybody loves chocolate, and this is perfect for the occasional treat. Good-quality chocolate tends to be lower in saturated fat than normal chocolate.

50g unsweetened plain cooking chocolate
  (minimum 70 per cent cocoa solids)
110g plain flour
110g caster sugar
1 tablespoon unsweetened cocoa powder
125ml skimmed milk
1 egg
1 teaspoon baking powder
½ teaspoon grated nutmeg
75g hazelnuts, toasted and chopped
Margarine, for greasing

Serves 6

Melt the chocolate in a bowl set over a saucepan of simmering water.

Combine the remaining ingredients, except for the hazelnuts, in a food processor or mixer and blend for 1 minute at low speed. Add the melted chocolate and blend for 1 minute at high speed. Fold in the hazelnuts.

Lightly grease a 1.2 litre pudding basin with margarine. Spoon the batter into the basin. Cover with a lid or a pleated greased sheet of foil tied securely with string.

Place the basin on a rack set in the bottom of a saucepan. Pour boiling water into the saucepan until it comes three-quarters of the way up the side of the basin. Cook over a medium heat for about 1½ hours or until a knife or skewer inserted into the centre of the pudding comes out clean.

Remove the pudding from the saucepan and allow to cool for 10 minutes. Run a knife around the edge to loosen and invert on to a serving dish. Serve with Vanilla Custard (see page 135).

PER SERVING:
289 KCALS, 13G FAT, 3G SATURATED FAT, 39G CARBOHYDRATE, 0.14G SODIUM

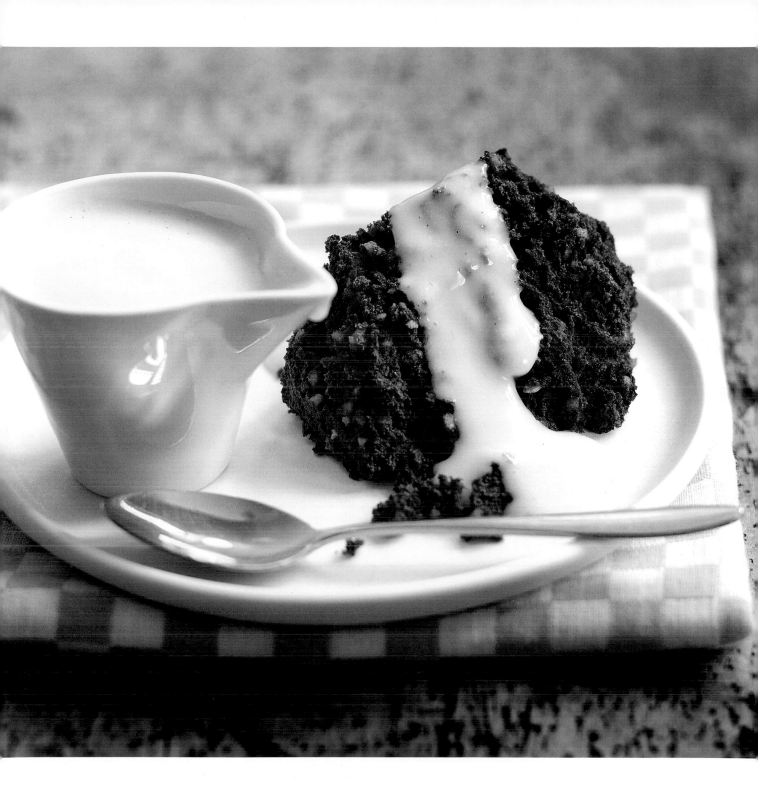

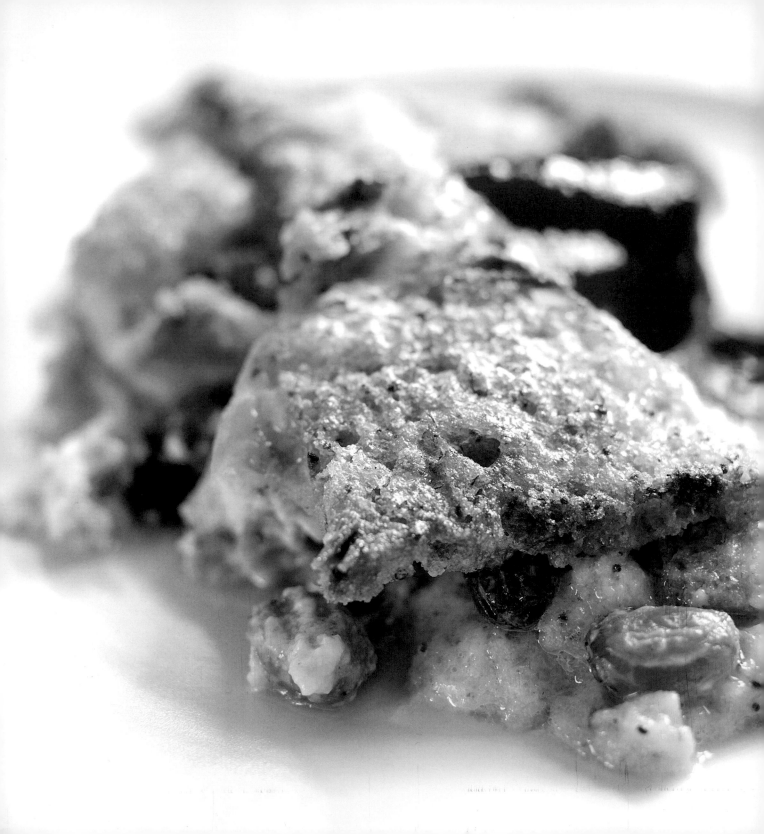

bread and butter pudding with raspberry sauce

Comfort food that we all need from time to time, this is a much-beloved recipe that is well worth the effort.

50g sultanas
50g raisins
4 tablespoons strong tea
1 tablespoon brandy extract or flavouring
14 slices medium-cut wholegrain bread
75g unsalted margarine, softened
4 eggs, plus 2 egg yolks
50g icing sugar
2 teaspoons vanilla extract
700ml skimmed milk
Pinch of grated nutmeg
2 tablespoons caster sugar

For the raspberry sauce
125g fresh raspberries
1 teaspoon icing sugar
Juice of 2 limes

Serves 8

Place the raisins and sultanas in a small non-metallic bowl and pour over the tea and the brandy extract. Cover with clingfilm and leave to soak for at least 2 hours (overnight is best). Drain off any excess juices and reserve.

Spread the bread with the margarine. Remove the crusts and cut each slice into 4 triangles. Grease a 2.5 litre shallow ovenproof dish with a little of the remaining margarine and arrange a layer of the bread triangles in the bottom of the dish, margarine-side up. Scatter over half of the soaked dried fruits and place another layer of the bread triangles on top, margarine-side up – you should have used about two-thirds of them at this stage. Set the remainder aside. Scatter over the remaining soaked dried fruits and press down gently into the dish with a fish slice.

Whisk together the eggs, egg yolks and the icing sugar in a large jug. Add the vanilla extract and milk, whisking to combine. Pour two-thirds of this custard over the layered bread triangles and leave to stand for 45 minutes–1 hour until the bread has soaked up all of the custard.

Preheat the oven to 180°C/350°F/gas mark 4.

Pour the remaining custard mixture over the soaked bread and margarine triangles. Arrange the rest of the bread triangles on top, margarine-side up. Press the slices down firmly with a fish slice so that the custard comes half-way up the bread triangles. Sprinkle over the nutmeg and caster sugar.

Place the dish into a roasting tin and pour warm water into the tin so that it comes three-quarters of the way up the dish. Bake for 35–40 minutes or until the custard has just set and the top is golden brown.

To make the sauce, place all the ingredients in a liquidiser and process until smooth. Pass through a fine sieve to remove the pips. Refrigerate until ready to serve.

Drizzle some raspberry sauce over the pudding and serve.

PER SERVING:
361 KCALS, 14G FAT, 4G SATURATED FAT, 49G CARBOHYDRATE, 0.47G SODIUM

index

resources

UK

Diabetes Research & Wellness Foundation
(DRWF)
The Roundhouse
010-012 Northney Marina
Hayling Island
HAMPSHIRE
PO11 0NH
www.drwf.org.uk
enquiries@drwf.org.uk
Tel: 023 92 637808

DRWF also has branches in
France (www.a-rd.fr), Sweden
(www.diabeteswellness.se) and
Finland (www.diabeteswellness.fi).

Diabetes UK
Macleod House
10 Parkway
London NW1 7AA
www.diabetes.org.uk
info@diabetes.org.uk
0345 123 2399

US

Diabetes Research & Wellness Foundation
(DRWF)
1832 Connecticut Ave, NW
Washington, DC 20009
www.diabeteswellness.net
Diabeteswellness@diabeteswellness.net
1 866 293-3155

Australia

Diabetes Australia
PO Box 3156
Canberra ACT 2607
www.diabetesaustralia.com.au
admin@diabetesaustralia.com.au
02 6232 3800

Canada

Canadian Diabetes Association
www.diabetes.ca
info@diabetes.ca
1800 226 8464

Acknowledgements

Writing this book has been a great
pleasure for me. This was made almost
effortless by the co-operation of Antony,
who tirelessly took on board the sometimes
challenging requests. I also have been
supported by Muna Reyal, who has been
understanding and obliging throughout.
Special people have shaped my
writing the inspirational life coach Nina
Puddefoot, dietitian and lecturer Sue Baic,
my husband Shamil and my children,
Shazia and Bizhan. Lastly, I would like to
acknowledge the trust which the Diabetes
Research and Wellness Foundation has
placed in me. AG

This revised edition published in Great Britain 2016
by Kyle Books, an imprint of Kyle Cathie Ltd.
192–198 Vauxhall Bridge Road
London, SW1V 1DX
general.enquiries@kylebooks.com
www.kylebooks.co.uk

First published 2003 by Kyle Cathie Ltd.

10 9 8 7 6 5 4 3 2 1

ISBN 978 0 85783 295 5

Antony Worrall Thompson and Azmina Govindji
are hereby identified as the authors of this work
in accordance with Section 77 of the Copyright,
Designs and Patents Act 1988.

Text © 2003 Antony Worrall Thompson
and Azmina Govindji
Photography © 2003 Steve Lee
Book design © 2003 Kyle Cathie Limited

Senior Editor Muna Reyal
Designer Carl Hodson
Photographer Steve Lee
Home economist Jane Suthering
Assistant to home economist Julian Biggs
Styling Penny Markham
Copyeditor Anne Newman
Recipe analysis Dr Wendy Doyle
Production Sha Huxtable

A Cataloguing In Publication record for this title is
available from the British Library.

Colour reproduction by Sang Choy
Printed and bound in China by C&C Offset
Printing Co., Ltd.

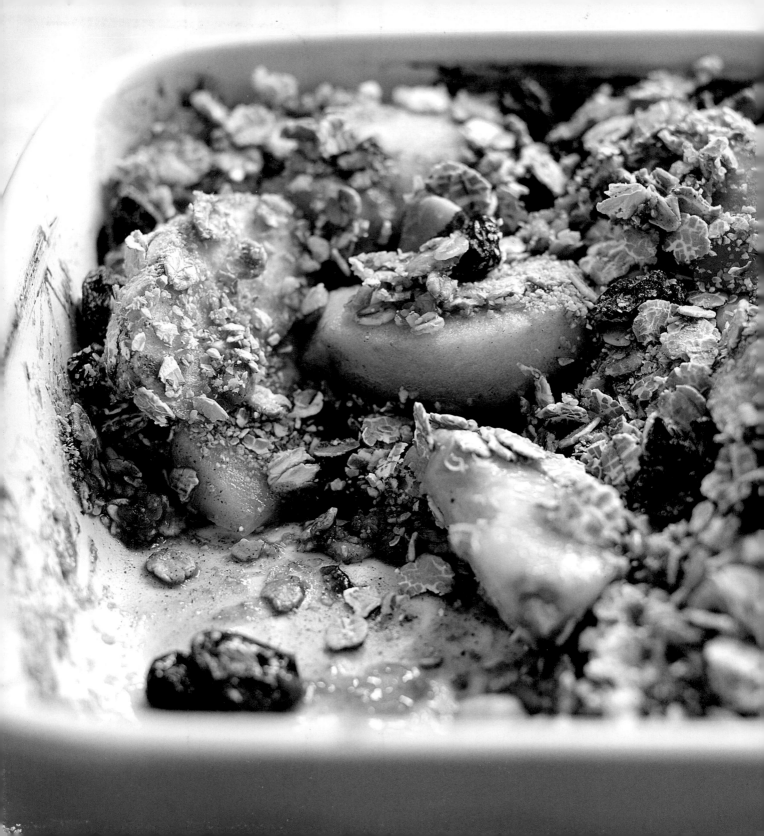